HANDBOOK FOR
Anesthesia and Co-Existing Disease

HANDBOOK FOR
Anesthesia and Co-Existing Disease

Robert K. Stoelting, M.D.
Professor and Chairman
Department of Anesthesia
Indiana University School of Medicine
Indianapolis, Indiana

Stephen F. Dierdorf, M.D.
Professor
Department of Anesthesia
Indiana University School of Medicine
Indianapolis, Indiana

Churchill Livingstone
New York, Edinburgh, London, Madrid, Melbourne, Tokyo

Library of Congress Cataloging-in-Publication Data

Handbook for Anesthesia and co-existing disease / [edited by] Robert
  K. Stoelting, Stephen F. Dierdorf.
        p.   cm.
    Includes bibliographical references and index.
    ISBN 0-443-08893-4
    1. Anesthesia—Complications—Handbooks, manuals, etc.
2. Therapeutics, Surgical—Handbooks, manuals, etc.   I. Stoelting,
Robert K. II. Dierdorf, Stephen F.   III. Anesthesia and co-existing
disease.
    [DNLM: 1. Anesthesia—adverse effects—outlines. 2. Anesthetics—
outlines. WO 245 A578 1993 Suppl.]
RD87.A53 1993 Suppl.
617.9'6041—dc20
DNLM/DLC
for Library of Congress   93-707
                                                               CIP

Distributed in the United Kingdom by Churchill Livingstone, Robert
Stevenson House, 1–3 Baxter's Place, Leith Walk, Edinburgh EH1 3AF,
and by associated companies, branches, and representatives throughout
the world.

Accurate indications, adverse reactions, and dosage schedules for drugs
are provided in this book, but it is possible that they may change. The
reader is urged to review the package information data of the manufac-
turers of the medications mentioned.

The Publishers have made every effort to trace the copyright holders for
borrowed material. If they have inadvertently overlooked any, they will be
pleased to make the necessary arrangements at the first opportunity.

Acquisitions Editor: *Toni M. Tracy*
Copy Editor: *Bridgett Dickinson*
Production Designer: *Susan Fung*
Production Supervisor: *Jeanine Furino*
Cover Design: *Paul Moran*

Printed in the United States of America

First published in 1993   7   6   5   4   3   2   1

Preface

The *Handbook for Anesthesia and Co-Existing Disease* is intended to provide a convenient and rapid source of information relevant to the impact of the pathophysiology of disease states on the perioperative management of patients. The Handbook uses an outline format that follows the identical chapters and headings in the third edition of *Anesthesia and Co-Existing Disease*, thus allowing the student and practitioner to refer to sources easily. As such, the intent is for the Handbook to serve as a bridge to *Anesthesia and Co-Existing Disease* and its more in-depth discussion of each disease entity. The emphasis in the Handbook is on presentation of information in table format. This design provides rapid visibility of pertinent aspects of a patient's medical condition that can be readily accessed, if needed, on-site in the operating room or other areas of the health care facility that are remote from the individual's personal library.

We wish to thank Deanna M. Walker for her secretarial help in the preparation of the manuscript. We also thank Toni M. Tracy, President of Churchill Livingstone, for her support of this new venture.

Robert K. Stoelting, M.D.
Stephen F. Dierdorf, M.D.

Contents

CHAPTER 1

Ischemic Heart Disease

Ischemic heart disease (IHD), which reflects the presence of atherosclerosis in coronary arteries (coronary artery disease), is estimated to be present in 10 million adult Americans (see Stoelting RK, Dierdorf SF. Ischemic heart disease. In: Anesthesia and Co-Existing Disease. 3rd Ed. New York. Churchill Livingstone, 1993). Among the estimated 25 million patients in the United States who undergo surgery each year, approximately 3 million have IHD.

I. RISK FACTORS

  A. The two most important risk factors for the development of atherosclerosis involving the coronary arteries are **male gender and increasing age** (Table 1-1). Three additional risk factors are **hypercholesterolemia, hypertension, and cigarette smoking.**

   1. There is a linear correlation between the plasma concentration of cholesterol and the risk of development of IHD (risk doubled in those with a plasma cholesterol level >240 mg·dl^{-1} compared with a level <180 mg·dl^{-1}).

   2. Hypertension may augment the risk of IHD by enhancing the process of arterial wall injury that leads to atherosclerosis. Nevertheless, control of hypertension is probably more important in preventing stroke than myocardial infarction.

   3. Cigarette smoking is estimated to be responsible for 30% of the 500,000 fatalities attributed to IHD.

      a. Addition of the risk factor of cigarette smoking is equivalent to increasing the plasma cholesterol concentration by 50 to 100 mg·dl^{-1}.

      b. The risk of IHD seems to be related to the concurrent level of smoking and to be reversible when smoking is discontinued.

II. CARDIAC EVALUATION

  A. History, physical examination, chest radiograph, and electrocardiogram (ECG) are the basic components of the cardiac evaluation and diagnosis of the patient with known or suspected IHD (Table 1-2).

Table 1-1. *Risk Factors for the Development of Ischemic Heart Disease*

Male gender
Increasing age
Hypercholesterolemia
Hypertension
Cigarette smoking
Diabetes mellitus
Obesity
Psychosocial characteristics
Sedentary life-style
Family history of premature development of ischemic heart disease

Table 1-2. *Diagnosis of Ischemic Heart Disease*

Initial Evaluation
   History
   Physical examination
   Laboratory data

Stress Testing If Initial Evaluation Suggestive
   Exercise electrocardiogram
   Radionuclide tests
      Exercise thallium
      Dipyridamole thallium

Stress Test Suggestive
   Coronary angiography

1. Specialized and expensive noninvasive and invasive tests are employed selectively as adjuncts to the basic components of the cardiac evaluation.
2. **Left ventricular function can be classified** as good or impaired on the basis of the cardiac evaluation (Table 1-3).

B. History
1. An important goal of the history is to elicit the severity, progression, and functional limitations introduced by IHD (Table 1-4).
2. **Cardiac dysrhythmias, myocardial ischemia, and left ventricular dysfunction** are usually responsible for symptoms of IHD.

Table 1-3. *Evaluation of Left Ventricular Function*

Good Function	Impaired Function
History and Physical Examination	
Angina pectoris	Prior myocardial infarction
Essential hypertension	Evidence of congestive heart
No evidence of congestive heart failure	failure
Cardiac Catheterization	
Ejection fraction >0.55	Ejection fraction <0.4
Left ventricular end-diastolic pressure <12 mmHg	Left ventricular end-diastolic pressure >18 mmHg
Cardiac index >2.5 L•min^{-1}•m^{-2}	Cardiac index <2 L•min^{-1}•m^{-2}
No areas of ventricular dyskinesia	Multiple areas of ventricular dyskinesia

Table 1-4. *Cardiac Evaluation by History*

Exercise tolerance (cardiac reserve likely to be adequate if patient can climb two to three flights of stairs without symptoms)

Angina pectoris

Prior myocardial infarction

Co-existing noncardiac diseases
  Peripheral vascular disease
  Chronic obstructive airway disease
  Renal dysfunction
  Diabetes mellitus

Current medications
  Beta antagonists
  Nitrates
  Calcium entry blockers
  Aspirin

3. **Dyspnea** following the onset of angina suggests the presence of acute left ventricular dysfunction (congestive heart failure [CHF]) due to myocardial ischemia. It is important to identify the patient bordering on CHF as the added stress of anesthesia, surgery, and fluid replacement may result in overt CHF.

4. **Angina pectoris is considered stable** when there has been no change in the precipitating factors, frequency, and duration of pain for at least 60 days.

5. Angina pectoris produced with less than normal activity or that lasts for more prolonged periods than experienced previously is considered characteristic of unstable angina and may signal impending myocardial infarction.

6. **Silent myocardial ischemia** does not evoke angina and usually occurs at a heart rate and blood pressure substantially lower than that present during exercise-induced myocardial ischemia. **It is estimated that about 70% of ischemic episodes in patients with symptomatic IHD are not associated with angina** and that about 10% to 15% of acute myocardial infarctions are silent.

7. **The incidence of myocardial reinfarction** during the perioperative period is related to the **time elapsed since the previous myocardial infarction.**

   a. The incidence of perioperative myocardial reinfarction seems to stabilize at about 6% (incidence is 0.13% in the absence of a prior myocardial infarction) after about 6 months (Table 1-5).

   b. This is the basis for the recommendation that an elective operation, especially a thoracic or upper abdomi-

Table 1-5. *Incidence of Perioperative Myocardial Reinfarction*

Time Elapsed Since Prior Myocardial Infarction (mo)	Tarhan et al[a] (%)	Steen et al[b] (%)	Rao et al[c] (%)	Shah et al[d] (%)
0–3	37	27	5.7	4.3
4–6	16	11	2.3	0
>6	5	6		5.7

[a] Tarhan S, Moffitt EA, Taylor WF, Guiliani ER. Myocardial infarction after general anesthesia. JAMA 1972;220:1451-4.
[b] Steen PA, Tinker JH, Tarhan S. Myocardial infarction after anesthesia and surgery. An update: Incidence, mortality, and predisposing factors. JAMA 1978;239:2566-70.
[c] Rao TLK, Jacobs KH, El-Etr AA. Reinfarction following anesthesia in patients with myocardial infarction. Anesthesiology 1983;59:499-505.
[d] Shah KB, Kleinman BS, Sami H, Patel J, Rao TLK. Reevaluation of perioperative myocardial infarction in patients with prior myocardial infarction undergoing noncardiac operations. Anesth Analg 1991;71:231-5.

nal procedure expected to last >3 hours, be delayed for about 6 months after a myocardial infarction.

    c. Mortality after myocardial reinfarction exceeds 20%; more than 90% of these adverse cardiac events occur within the first 48 hours after operation.

    d. The risk of postoperative myocardial infarction after noncardiac surgery is increased in the patient with known three-vessel coronary artery disease and in those with left main coronary artery disease.

  8. Medical therapy for IHD is designed to decrease myocardial oxygen requirements and to improve coronary blood flow. These goals are most often achieved by the combined use of a beta antagonist, nitrate, and calcium entry blocker.

    a. Effective beta blockade is probably present when the resting heart rate is 50 to 60 beats·min^{-1}.

    b. The postoperative period is a time when inadvertent acute withdrawal of beta antagonist therapy may occur, resulting in rebound increases in blood pressure and heart rate.

    c. Transdermal preparations of nitroglycerin provide a sustained therapeutic effect.

    d. Treatment of a patient with a calcium entry blocker may introduce the potential **for adverse drug interactions** (e.g., volatile anesthetics, muscle relaxants, beta antagonists) during the perioperative period.

C. Physical Examination

  1. Signs of left ventricular failure should be detected preoperatively.

  2. Orthostatic hypotension may reflect attenuated autonomic nervous system activity due to treatment with an antihypertensive drug.

  3. The physical examination is often normal despite significant IHD.

D. Chest Radiograph. Evidence of cardiomegaly and CHF is routinely sought.

E. Electrocardiogram

  1. Review of the ECG is a cost-effective screening test in the cardiac evaluation of a patient with IHD (Table 1-6).

  2. The resting ECG in the absence of angina may be normal despite extensive IHD.

  3. The accepted criterion for an ischemic response on the resting or exercise ECG is ST segment depression of

---

Table 1-6. *Cardiac Evaluation and Information Available from the Electrocardiogram*

Myocardial ischemia

Prior myocardial infarction

Cardiac rhythm and/or conduction disturbances

Cardiomegaly

Electrolyte abnormalities

---

1 mm or more in a patient in whom the ST segments were previously isoelectric.

   a. The ECG lead demonstrating ST segment depression can help determine the specific coronary artery that is diseased (Table 1-7).

   b. The exercise ECG **simulates sympathetic nervous system stimulation** that may accompany perioperative events such as laryngoscopy and surgical stimulation.

   c. **Vasospastic angina** is characterized by ST segment elevation on the ECG during periods of myocardial ischemia.

   F. Advanced diagnostic methods as used in the cardiac evaluation of the patient with suspected IHD may be categorized as noninvasive and invasive (Table 1-8).

Table 1-7. *Relationship of the Electrocardiogram Lead to the Area of Myocardial Ischemia*

Electrocardiogram Lead	Coronary Artery Branch Responsible for Ischemia	Area of Myocardium That May Be Involved
II, III, aVF	Right coronary artery	Right atrium Right ventricle Sinoatrial node Atrioventricular node
I, aVL	Circumflex coronary artery	Lateral aspects of left ventricle
V3–V5	Left anterior descending coronary artery	Anterolateral aspects of left ventricle

Table 1-8. *Advanced Diagnostic Methods in Cardiac Evaluation*

Ambulatory electrocardiographic monitoring (detect cardiac dysrhythmias)

Echocardiography (wall motion, cavity dimensions, valve function, ejection fraction)

Radioisotope imaging

Thallium scan (visualize blood flow to left ventricle; constant flow defect reflects old myocardial infarction, whereas exercise-induced flow defect reflects myocardial ischemia)

Radionuclide angiocardiography with technetium (images blood in heart and lungs; indicates contractility, areas of dyskinesia; used for calculation of ejection fraction)

Angiography

Coronary angiography (digital subtraction angiography; reflects condition of the coronary arteries; mortality 0.1%)

Left ventricular angiography (calculation of ejection fraction and evaluation of contractility)

Cardiac catheterization (left ventricular end-diastolic pressure <12 mmHg; cardiac index >2.5 $L \cdot min^{-1} \cdot m^{-2}$)

III. ACUTE MYOCARDIAL INFARCTION

A. **Diagnosis** of myocardial infarction is based on the onset of characteristic symptoms (e.g., angina pectoris unrelieved by nitroglycerin, ventricular premature beats, hypotension) followed by serial ECG changes (ST and T wave changes, Q waves) and transient increases in the plasma concentration of myocardial enzymes (CK-MB increases at least 50% during first 4 to 12 hours).

1. Myocardial infarction may be silent, although the development of cardiac dysrhythmias, hypotension, or CHF during the perioperative period should arouse suspicion.

2. Myocardial infarction that occurs during the perioperative period may be difficult to recognize because of concurrent medical circumstances such as operation-related pain and administration of analgesics.

B. **Treatment** of an acute myocardial infarction is both medical and surgical (Table 1-9).

Table 1-9. *Treatment of an Acute Myocardial Infarction*

Thrombolytic therapy (institute within 6 hours; intracranial hemorrhage a risk and reocclusion occurs in about 20% of treated patients)

Beta antagonist (may decrease infarct size and incidence of reinfarction)

Lidocaine (decreases incidence of cardiac dysrhythmias)

Artificial cardiac pacemaker

Emergency coronary arteriography and percutaneous transluminal coronary angioplasty (PTCA)

Table 1-10. *Complications of an Acute Myocardial Infarction*

Cardiac dysrhythmias and conduction disturbances (premature ventricular beats occur in >90% of patients; bradycardia)

Pericarditis

Pericardial effusion

Left ventricular thrombus

Congestive heart failure

Cardiogenic shock (an advanced form of congestive heart failure; systolic blood pressure often <60 mmHg in presence of pulmonary edema and arterial hypoxemia; treatment is with inotropes, circulatory assist devices)

Ventricular septal rupture

Acute mitral regurgitation

Ventricular aneurysm

Cardiac rupture

    C. Complications following an acute myocardial infarction may be life-threatening or rapidly fatal (Table 1-10).

IV. ANESTHESIA FOR NONCARDIAC SURGERY (see also section II, Cardiac Evaluation)

    A. Preoperative Medication

        1. The goal of preoperative medication for the patient with IHD is to **decrease anxiety.** This is because activation of the sympathetic nervous system may increase myocardial

oxygen requirements and evoke myocardial ischemia.
2. Maximum sedation and amnesia without an undesirable degree of circulatory and ventilatory depression may be achieved with scopolamine and a benzodiazepine.
   a. Nitroglycerin ointment may be applied at the same time that the preoperative medication is administered.
   b. Drugs used in the medical management of a patient with IHD should be continued throughout the perioperative period, including, in some instances, administration of these drugs with the preoperative medication.

B. Intraoperative Management
1. The basic challenge during induction and maintenance of anesthesia is to prevent intraoperative events that will adversely alter the balance between myocardial oxygen delivery and myocardial oxygen requirements, predisposing the patient to the development of myocardial ischemia (Table 1-11).
   a. A frequent recommendation is to maintain heart rate and blood pressure within 20% of the normal awake value for that patient.
   b. An increase in heart rate (particularly >110

Table 1-11. *Intraoperative Events That Influence the Balance Between Myocardial Oxygen Delivery and Myocardial Oxygen Requirements*

Decreased Oxygen Delivery	Increased Oxygen Requirements
Decreased coronary blood flow	Sympathetic nervous
Tachycardia	system stimulation
Diastolic hypotension	Tachycardia
Hypocapnia (coronary	Systolic hypertension
vasoconstriction)	Increased myocardial
Coronary artery spasm	contractility
	Increased afterload
Decreased oxygen content	
Anemia	
Arterial hypoxemia	
Shift of the oxyhemoglobin	
dissociation curve to the left	
Increased preload (wall tension)	

beats·min^{-1}) is more likely than hypertension to produce signs of myocardial ischemia recorded on the ECG (Fig. 1-1).

   c. Despite appropriate precautions, most episodes of intraoperative myocardial ischemia recorded on the ECG occur in the absence of hemodynamic changes. It is therefore unlikely that this "silent myocardial ischemia" can be prevented by the anesthesiologist.

   d. Perioperative episodes of silent myocardial ischemia are most likely identical to episodes that occur in these patients during their daily activity in the absence of angina. They are therefore of doubtful significance.

C. Induction of anesthesia in the patient with IHD can be accomplished with most of the currently available intravenous induction drugs. However, ketamine is not popu-

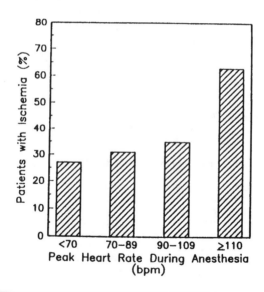

Fig. 1-1. *The incidence of intraoperative myocardial ischemia is unrelated to heart rate (silent ischemia), until the heart rate exceeds about 110 beats · min^{-1} (bpm). (From Slogoff S, Keats AS. Does chronic treatment with calcium entry blocking drugs reduce perioperative myocardial ischemia? Anesthesiology 1988;68:676–80, with permission.)*

lar, since an associated increase in heart rate and blood pressure might increase myocardial oxygen requirements.

1. Myocardial ischemia may accompany sympathetic nervous system stimulation that results from direct laryngoscopy and intubation of the trachea.

   a. **A short duration of laryngoscopy** (<15 seconds) may be useful in minimizing the magnitude and duration of circulatory stimulation associated with intubation of the trachea.

   b. When the duration of direct laryngoscopy is not likely to be short, or when hypertension already exists, it is reasonable to consider the use of additional drugs to minimize the blood pressure and/or heart rate response produced by the intubation sequence (Table 1-12).

D. **Maintenance of anesthesia** in the patient with IHD is often accomplished with drugs chosen on the basis of the patient's left ventricular function, as determined by the history and physical examination, with or without data from cardiac catheterization (Table 1-3).

   1. In the presence of normal left ventricular function, **controlled myocardial depression** using a volatile anesthetic may be appropriate so as to minimize increased sympathetic nervous system activity and increased myocardial oxygen requirements.

Table 1-12. *Drugs Intended to Attenuate the Blood Pressure and/or Heart Rate Response to Tracheal Intubation*

Laryngotracheal lidocaine

Lidocaine (1.5 mg•kg^{-1} IV 90 seconds before beginning direct laryngoscopy)

Nitroprusside (1–2 µg•kg^{-1} IV 15 seconds before beginning direct laryngoscopy)

Esmolol (100–300 µg•kg^{-1}•min^{-1} IV before and during direct laryngoscopy)

Fentanyl (1–3 µg•kg^{-1} IV administered before direct laryngoscopy)

Nitroglycerin (0.25–1 µg•kg^{-1}•min^{-1} IV) to decrease the pressor response (but no evidence that the incidence of intraoperative myocardial ischemia is decreased)

    a. Volatile anesthetics, with or without nitrous oxide, are equally acceptable to produce controlled myocardial depression (Fig. 1-2).

    b. An alternative to a volatile anesthetic is a nitrous oxide–opioid combination with the addition of a volatile anesthetic to treat an undesirable increase in blood pressure that may accompany painful stimulation.

    c. Despite the ability of isoflurane to cause coronary artery vasodilation (**coronary artery steal**), there is no evidence that this drug increases the likelihood of myocardial ischemia.

2. High-dose fentanyl (50 to 100 $\mu g \cdot kg^{-1}$ IV, or an equivalent dose of sufentanil) has been recommended for patients who cannot tolerate even minimal drug-induced myocardial depression.

3. Choice of muscle relaxant is influenced by the impact these drugs could have on the balance between myocardial oxygen delivery and requirements.

    a. Vecuronium, doxacurium, and pipecuronium are examples of drugs with benign circulatory effects.

    b. Pancuronium has the ability to increase myocardial oxygen requirements by virtue of drug-induced increases in heart rate and blood pressure.

    c. Reversal of nondepolarizing neuromuscular blockade with an anticholinesterase–anticholinergic drug combination can be safely accomplished in a patient with IHD.

4. Monitoring is influenced by the complexity of the operative procedure and by the severity of the IHD.

    a. Important goals in selecting monitors uniquely for the patient with IHD are detection of myocardial ischemia (ECG), recognition of decreased myocardial contractility (pulmonary artery catheter, transesophageal echocardiography), and evaluation of the intravascular fluid volume (pulmonary artery catheter, central venous pressure).

    b. An acute increase in the pulmonary artery occlusion pressure associated with the appearance of an abnormal A wave or V wave may reflect the presence of myocardial ischemia.

    c. Appearance of signs of myocardial ischemia on the ECG supports prompt and aggressive pharmacologic

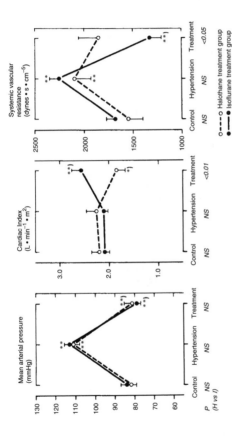

Fig. 1-2. Halothane (1% to 1.5% inspired) and isoflurane (1.5% to 2% inspired) were equally effective in returning mean arterial pressure to near-control levels in patients who became hypertensive during surgical revascularization of the coronary circulation. Halothane lowers blood pressure principally by decreasing myocardial contractility (cardiac index), whereas decreased blood pressure produced by isoflurane is due principally to decreased systemic vascular resistance. (From Hess W, Arnold B, Schulte-Sasse U, Tarnow J. Comparison of isoflurane and halothane when used to control intraoperative hypertension in patients undergoing coronary artery bypass surgery. Anesth Analg 1983;62:15–20, with permission.)

Table 1-13. *Treatment of Myocardial Ischemia As Evidenced on the Electrocardiogram*

Esmolol if heart rate is increased

Nitroglycerin if blood pressure is normal or elevated (nitroprusside a consideration if blood pressure is elevated in absence of myocardial ischemia)

Sympathomimetic drug if blood pressure is decreased (ephedrine and phenylephrine appear equally acceptable)

Intravenous fluids if blood pressure is decreased (unlike a sympathomimetic, may not be promptly effective)

treatment of associated adverse changes in heart rate and/or blood pressure (Table 1-13).
   d. The central venous pressure and pulmonary artery occlusion pressure are more likely to correlate when the ejection fraction is >0.5.
   e. Transesophageal echocardiography permits continuous intraoperative assessment of left ventricular function, especially when the surgical procedure includes cross-clamping of the aorta.
   5. In the final analysis, maintenance of the balance between myocardial oxygen requirements and myocardial oxygen delivery is probably more important than the specific technique or drugs chosen to produce anesthesia and skeletal muscle relaxation.
E. Postoperative Period. Pain-induced activation of the sympathetic nervous system may lead to increased myocardial oxygen requirements and myocardial ischemia, emphasizing the unique importance of providing adequate postoperative pain relief to the patient with IHD.

V. HEART TRANSPLANTATION

A. Preoperatively the ejection fraction is typically <0.2.
B. Management of Anesthesia
   1. Induction of anesthesia may include ketamine or a benzodiazepam plus an opioid for analgesia during surgery. Alternatively, an opioid may be used alone for induction and maintenance of anesthesia.

2. Nitrous oxide is seldom used because of additive depressant effects in the presence of opioids and concern about enlargement of an accidental air embolus that may occur when large blood vessels are opened during the operation.

3. Airway equipment and the anesthetic delivery tubing are maintained sterile, and bacterial filters are often used.

   a. Immunosuppressive drugs are usually initiated during the preoperative period.

   b. Intravascular catheters are placed using an aseptic technique. A central venous catheter or pulmonary artery catheter must be withdrawn back into the internal jugular vein during removal of the recipient's heart.

   c. Utilization of the left internal jugular vein for catheter placement preserves the right internal jugular vein as an access site to perform cardiac biopsies during the postoperative period.

4. Coagulopathy may reflect passive congestion of the liver due to chronic CHF.

5. An inotropic drug, especially isoproterenol, may be needed briefly to maintain myocardial contractility and heart rate (denervated transplanted heart initially assumes an intrinsic heart rate of about 110 beats·min^{-1}) of the donor heart after cardiopulmonary bypass.

6. Therapeutic attempts to lower pulmonary vascular resistance may be necessary, including administration of isoproterenol and vasodilating prostaglandin preparations.

C. Complications

1. Early postoperative morbidity is linked to surgical complications (hemorrhage), opportunistic infection, and rejection (evidenced on endomyocardial biopsy and by CHF).

2. Sympathetic nervous system reinnervation may occur within 6 to 12 months, manifesting in some transplant patients as angina pectoris.

3. Cyclosporine-induced hypertension and nephrotoxicity are possible side effects.

CHAPTER 2

Valvular Heart Disease

The most frequently encountered cardiac valve lesions produce pressure overload (mitral stenosis, aortic stenosis) or volume overload (mitral regurgitation, aortic regurgitation) on the left atrium or left ventricle (see Stoelting RK, Dierdorf SF. Valvular heart disease. In: Anesthesia and Co-Existing Disease. 3rd Ed. New York. Churchill Livingstone, 1993). Drug selections during the perioperative period for the patient with valvular heart disease are based on the likely effects that a drug-induced change in cardiac rhythm, heart rate (HR), blood pressure (BP), systemic vascular resistance (SVR), and pulmonary vascular resistance (PVR) will have relative to the pathophysiology of the heart disease.

I. PREOPERATIVE EVALUATION

A. History and Physical Examination

1. Preoperative evaluation of the patient with valvular heart disease includes assessment of the (1) severity of the cardiac disease, (2) degree of impaired myocardial contractility, (3) presence of associated major organ disease (pulmonary, renal, hepatic), and (4) development of compensatory mechanisms for maintaining cardiac output (increased sympathetic nervous system activity, cardiac hypertrophy).

   a. **Exercise tolerance** is useful for evaluating cardiac reserve and classifying the patient with valvular heart disease (Table 2-1).

   b. **Congestive heart failure (CHF),** manifesting as dyspnea, orthopnea, and fatigue, is a frequent companion of chronic valvular heart disease (see Chapter 6). Ideally, elective surgery is deferred until CHF can be treated and myocardial contractility optimized.

   c. **Anxiety, diaphoresis, and resting tachycardia** may reflect a compensatory increase in sympathetic nervous system activity.

   d. The character, location, intensity, and direction of radiation of the heart murmur provide a clue as to the location and severity of the cardiac valve lesion (Fig. 2-1).

   e. **Cardiac dysrhythmias,** especially **atrial fibrillation,** are common.

Table 2-1. *New York Heart Association Classification of Patients With Heart Disease*

Class	Description
I	Asymptomatic
II	Symptoms with ordinary activity but comfortable at rest
III	Symptoms with minimal activity but comfortable at rest
IV	Symptoms at rest

   f. Angina pectoris may be due to increased cardiac muscle mass that exceeds the ability of even normal coronary arteries to deliver adequate amounts of oxygen.
2. Preoperative evaluation of the patient with a **prosthetic heart valve** includes (1) evaluation for paravalvular leak or other mechanical dysfunction, (2) determination of the presence of CHF, and (3) management of anticoagulation.
   a. Changes in cardiac valve sounds or the appearance of a new heart murmur are sought.
   b. An increased incidence of cholecystitis may reflect chronic low-grade intravascular hemolysis.

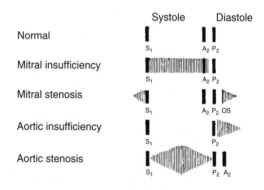

Fig. 2-1. Timing and characteristics of cardiac murmurs in relationship to systole and diastole. (From Fishman MC, Hoffman AR, Klausner RD, Rockson SG, Thaler MS. Medicine. Philadelphia. JB Lippincott 1984;42, with permission.)

B. **Drug Therapy**
   1. **Digitalis** is most often administered to increase myocardial contractility and to slow the ventricular HR response in the patient with atrial fibrillation.
      a. **An adequate digitalis effect** for HR control is indicated by a ventricular rate of <80 beats·min^{-1} at rest.
      b. **Digitalis toxicity** is suggested by prolongation of the P-R interval and appearance of ventricular premature beats on the electrocardiogram (ECG).
   2. **Diuretic therapy** is useful for treatment of excess intravascular fluid volume but may result in total body potassium depletion and vulnerability to the development of digitalis toxicity.

C. **Laboratory Data**
   1. **Doppler echocardiography** has revolutionized the noninvasive evaluation of valvular heart disease (Table 2-2).
   2. **Cardiac catheterization** provides useful information (cardiac filling pressures, transvalvular pressure gradient) as to the severity of valvular heart disease.
   3. **Arterial blood gases** may reflect a decrease in PaO$_2$, most likely owing to interstitial pulmonary edema and altered ventilation-to-perfusion relationships.

D. **Treatment**
   1. Although commissurotomy may be considered, the only effective therapy for most patients is replacement of the damaged valve with a prosthetic valve.
   2. The greatest disadvantage of a prosthetic heart valve is its tendency to promote thrombus formation and the subsequent risk of systemic embolization.

Table 2-2. *Doppler Echocardiography and Valvular Heart Disease*

Determine significance of cardiac murmurs (most often aortic stenosis)

Identify hemodynamic abnormalities associated with physical findings (most often mitral regurgitation)

Determine transvalvular pressure gradient

Determine orifice area of cardiac valve

Diagnose cardiac valve regurgitation

Evaluate prosthetic valve function

II. MITRAL STENOSIS

A. Pathophysiology

1. Mitral stenosis is almost always due to fusion of the mitral valve leaflets at the commissures during the healing process of acute rheumatic fever.

2. Measurement of the diastolic pressure gradient across the valve at cardiac catheterization provides the most definitive assessment of the degree of mitral stenosis, with a gradient >10 mmHg (normal <5 mmHg) suggesting severe stenosis.

3. When the mitral valve area is <1 cm^2 (normal 4 to 6 cm^2), a mean left atrial pressure of about 25 mmHg is necessary to maintain an adequate resting cardiac output.

   a. **Interstitial or overt pulmonary edema** is possible when pulmonary venous pressure is increased as a result of increased left atrial pressure.

   b. **Pulmonary hypertension** is likely when the left atrial pressure is chronically >25 mmHg.

4. **Left atrial enlargement** predisposes to **atrial fibrillation.**

   a. Stasis of blood in the distended left atrium predisposes to the formation of thrombi, which can be displaced as systemic emboli, especially with the onset of atrial fibrillation.

   b. For these reasons, the patient with mitral stenosis may be receiving chronic anticoagulant therapy.

B. Management of Anesthesia

1. An important goal is to avoid events that may further decrease the cardiac output (Table 2-3).

   a. Treatment of rapid atrial fibrillation is cardioversion or an intravenous infusion of esmolol. Digoxin is useful when prolonged, but not immediate, control of HR is desirable.

   b. Treatment of a sudden decrease in SVR is with ephedrine or phenylephrine.

   c. Treatment of pulmonary hypertension and right ventricular failure may include inotropic support with dopamine and pulmonary vasodilation with nitroprusside.

2. **Preoperative medication** is intended to decrease the likelihood of anxiety-induced tachycardia.

   a. These patients may be more susceptible than a normal person to the ventilatory depressant effects of sedative drugs.

Table 2-3. *Anesthetic Considerations in the Patient With Mitral Stenosis*

Avoid sinus tachycardia or rapid ventricular response rate during atrial fibrillation

Avoid marked increases in central blood volume as associated with overtransfusion or head-down position

Avoid drug-induced decreases in systemic vascular resistance

Avoid events such as arterial hypoxemia and/or hypoventilation that may exacerbate pulmonary hypertension and evoke right ventricular failure

    b. Use of an anticholinergic drug is controversial because of concern that an adverse increase in HR could occur.

    c. **Prophylactic antibiotics** are recommended for protection against the development of infective endocarditis.

    d. The patient taking digitalis for control of the ventricular HR response during atrial fibrillation should have this drug continued until the time of surgery.

    e. Advisability of discontinuing anticoagulant medication before elective surgery is unclear.

3. **Induction of anesthesia** is most often accomplished with drugs administered intravenously that are unlikely to increase HR (avoid ketamine) or abruptly decrease SVR.

    a. There is no evidence that succinylcholine increases the incidence of ventricular dysrhythmias in patients being treated with digitalis.

    b. Pancuronium is an unlikely selection because of its ability to increase HR, which may be accentuated in the patient with atrial fibrillation.

4. **Maintenance of anesthesia** is intended to minimize the likelihood of marked and sustained changes in HR, SVR, PVR, and myocardial contractility.

    a. These goals are most likely to be achieved with the combination of nitrous oxide and an opioid or a low concentration of volatile drug.

    b. Nitrous oxide may increase PVR, especially in the presence of co-existing severe pulmonary hypertension.

   c. Nitroprusside-induced decreases in SVR may improve cardiac output in selected patients.

   d. Use of invasive monitoring depends on the complexity of the operative procedure and the magnitude of physiologic impairment produced by mitral stenosis. An asymptomatic patient without evidence of pulmonary congestion probably does not require monitoring different from the patient without valvular heart disease.

5. **Postoperatively** there is a risk of the development of pulmonary edema and right ventricular failure.

   a. Continuation of cardiac monitoring is indicated in selected patients.

   b. Mechanical support of ventilation may need to be continued, especially after major thoracic or abdominal surgery.

III. MITRAL REGURGITATION

A. Pathophysiology

1. Mitral regurgitation is usually due to rheumatic fever and is almost always associated with mitral stenosis.

2. Isolated mitral regurgitation in the absence of prior rheumatic fever is often acute (papillary muscle dysfunction after a myocardial infarction, rupture of a chordae tendineae secondary to infective endocarditis) or due to dilation of the mitral valve annulus owing to left ventricular hypertrophy.

3. Left atrial volume overload caused by retrograde flow of a portion of the left ventricular stroke volume into the left atrium is the principal pathophysiologic change produced by mitral regurgitation.

   a. Regurgitant flow is responsible for the V wave present on the recording of the pulmonary artery occlusion pressure (PAOP).

   b. The size of the V wave correlates with the magnitude of the regurgitant flow.

B. Management of Anesthesia

1. An important goal is to avoid events that may further decrease cardiac output (Table 2-4).

   a. Forward left ventricular stroke volume is facilitated by a modest increase in HR and decrease in SVR.

   b. Because left ventricular dysfunction usually accom-

Table 2-4. *Anesthetic Considerations in the Patient With Mitral Regurgitation*

Avoid sudden decreases in heart rate

Avoid sudden increases in systemic vascular resistance

Minimize drug-induced myocardial depression

Monitor the size of the V wave as a reflection of regurgitant flow

panies mitral regurgitation, even minimal drug-induced myocardial depression may be undesirable.

c. Drug-induced afterload reduction with nitroprusside combined with a cardiac inotrope such as dopamine may be useful for improving forward left ventricular stroke volume.

2. **Prophylactic antibiotics** are recommended for protection against the development of infective endocarditis.

3. **Induction of anesthesia** is most often accomplished with drugs administered intravenously, keeping in mind the importance of avoiding excessive and abrupt changes in SVR or decreases in HR (succinylcholine).

4. **Maintenance of anesthesia** is influenced by the degree of left ventricular dysfunction.

a. In the absence of severe left ventricular dysfunction, maintenance of anesthesia is often provided with nitrous oxide plus a volatile anesthetic (isoflurane is an attractive choice because of its hemodynamic effects).

b. When left ventricular dysfunction is severe, the use of an opioid technique that minimizes the likelihood of drug-induced myocardial depression may be a consideration.

c. Pancuronium is an attractive muscle relaxant selection because of the usually modest increase in HR produced by this drug.

d. Use of invasive monitoring depends on the complexity of the operative procedure and the magnitude of the physiologic impairment produced by mitral regurgitation. A pulmonary artery catheter is useful for monitoring the response to peripheral vasodilating drugs (change in V wave amplitude).

e. Maintenance of intravascular fluid volume with prompt replacement of blood loss is important for maintaining forward left ventricular stroke volume.

IV. MITRAL VALVE PROLAPSE

A. **Mitral valve prolapse** (prolapse of the mitral valve leaflets into the left atrium during systole) is the most common form of valvular heart disease, occurring in 5% to 10% of the general population (diagnosed most reliably by echocardiography).

B. **Complications** of mitral valve prolapse are usually benign but, on occasion, may be life-threatening (Table 2-5).

C. **Management of anesthesia** includes those principles outlined for the patient with mitral regurgitation (Table 2-4).

1. Increased left ventricular emptying (increased sympathetic nervous system activity, decreased SVR) can accentuate mitral valve prolapse, leading to cardiac dysrhythmias and/or acute mitral regurgitation.

2. **Prophylactic antibiotics** are recommended for protection against the development of infective endocarditis.

3. **Induction of anesthesia** can be achieved with available intravenous drugs, keeping in mind the need to avoid sudden and prolonged decreases in SVR and increases in sympathetic nervous system activity (ketamine may be avoided).

4. **Maintenance of anesthesia** is most often achieved with a volatile anesthetic combined with nitrous oxide and/or an opioid. Sudden and prolonged decreases in SVR (e.g., with epidural or spinal anesthesia) and increases in sympathetic nervous system activity should be avoided.

Table 2-5. *Complications Associated With Mitral Valve Prolapse*

Mitral regurgitation
Infective endocarditis
Ruptured chordae tendineae
Transient ischemic attack
Cardiac dysrhythmias—ventricular premature beats
Atrioventricular heart block
ST segment and T wave changes on the electrocardiogram
Sudden death (rare)

a. Titration of the volatile anesthetic is useful for minimizing sympathetic nervous system activation secondary to painful intraoperative stimulation.

b. Skeletal muscle paralysis is often provided with a nondepolarizing muscle relaxant that lacks significant circulatory effects (pancuronium may be avoided).

c. **Cardiac dysrhythmias** may occur unexpectedly, especially during an operation performed in the head-up or sitting position.

d. Prompt replacement of blood loss and generous intravenous fluid maintenance is useful for maintaining forward left ventricular stroke volume should acute mitral regurgitation occur intraoperatively.

V. AORTIC STENOSIS

A. Pathophysiology

1. Isolated nonrheumatic aortic stenosis usually results from progressive calcification and stenosis of a congenitally abnormal bicuspid valve, whereas aortic stenosis due to rheumatic fever almost always occurs in association with mitral valve disease.

2. Hemodynamically significant aortic stenosis is normally associated with a transvalvular pressure gradient >50 mmHg and an aortic valve orifice area <1 cm^2 (normal 2.5 to 3.5 cm^2).

3. The characteristic **triad** of symptoms associated with aortic stenosis includes angina pectoris (often in the absence of ischemic heart disease), dyspnea on exertion, and a history of syncope.

   a. The incidence of sudden death is increased in the patient with aortic stenosis.

   b. Since many patients with aortic stenosis are asymptomatic, it is important to listen for this heart murmur in patients scheduled for surgery.

B. Management of Anesthesia

1. An important goal is to avoid events that would further decrease cardiac output (Table 2-6).

2. **Prophylactic antibiotics** are recommended for protection against the development of infective endocarditis.

3. General anesthesia is often selected in preference to epidural anesthesia or spinal anesthesia to minimize the likelihood of an undesirable decrease in SVR.

Table 2-6. *Anesthetic Considerations in the Patient With Aortic Stenosis*

Maintain normal sinus rhythm
Avoid bradycardia
Avoid sudden increases or decreases in systemic vascular resis tance
Optimize intravascular fluid volume to maintain venous return and left ventricular filling

---

  a. Decreased SVR produced by isoflurane would be undesirable, although low concentrations of this anesthetic have not been recognized to be a hazard.
  b. Depression of sinoatrial node automaticity by a volatile anesthetic may lead to junctional rhythm, requiring prompt treatment with intravenous administration of atropine.
  c. When left ventricular function is severely impaired by aortic stenosis, it is useful to avoid any additional depression of myocardial contractility with a volatile anesthetic (opioids alone may be selected).
  d. Intravascular fluid volume is maintained by prompt replacement of blood loss and liberal administration of intravenous fluids.
 4. Use of an arterial and pulmonary artery catheter depends on the magnitude of the surgery and the severity of the aortic stenosis.
  a. These monitors help determine whether intraoperative hypotension is due to hypovolemia or CHF.
  b. The PAOP may overestimate left ventricular end-diastolic pressure because of decreased compliance of the left ventricle that accompanies aortic stenosis.

VI. AORTIC REGURGITATION

A. Pathophysiology

 1. Aortic regurgitation may be acute (infective endocarditis, trauma, dissection of a thoracic aneurysm) or chronic (prior rheumatic fever, persistent systemic hypertension).
 2. The basic hemodynamic problem in aortic regurgitation is a decrease in forward left ventricular stroke volume because of regurgitation of part of the ejected stroke volume from the aorta back into the left ventricle.

a. The magnitude of aortic regurgitation will be decreased by an increase in HR and a decrease in SVR.

b. An intravenous infusion of nitroprusside may be useful in improving forward left ventricular stroke volume when aortic regurgitation results in left ventricular volume overload and a decrease in cardiac output.

B. Management of Anesthesia

1. An important goal is to maintain forward left ventricular stroke volume (Table 2-7).

a. Overall a slight increase in HR and a modest decrease in SVR are desirable, recognizing that these patients may be exquisitely sensitive to peripheral vasodilation.

b. Left ventricular failure may be treated with afterload reduction, provided by nitroprusside and a cardiac inotrope (dopamine) to increase myocardial contractility.

2. **Prophylactic antibiotics** are recommended for protection against the development of infective endocarditis.

3. **General anesthesia** is often selected in preference to epidural anesthesia or spinal anesthesia, recognizing that desirable decreases in SVR produced by regional anesthesia may also be uncontrollable and unpredictable.

4. **Induction of anesthesia** is with drugs considered likely to maintain forward left ventricular stroke volume.

a. Ketamine is useful when intravascular fluid volume is decreased, recognizing that an excessive increase in SVR would be undesirable.

b. Bradycardia produced by succinylcholine is undesirable.

5. **Maintenance of anesthesia** in the absence of severe left ventricular dysfunction is often provided with nitrous oxide plus a volatile anesthetic (isoflurane is an attractive choice because of its hemodynamic effects) or an opioid.

Table 2-7. *Anesthetic Considerations in the Patient With Aortic Regurgitation*

Avoid sudden decreases in heart rate
Avoid sudden increases in systemic vascular resistance
Minimize drug-induced myocardial depression

    a. When myocardial function is compromised, the use of an opioid alone may be considered.

    b. Muscle relaxant selection may favor drugs with minimal to absent hemodynamic effects, although the modest increase in HR associated with pancuronium could contribute to the maintenance of forward left ventricular stroke volume.

    c. Maintenance of intravascular fluid volume with prompt replacement of blood loss is important for maintaining forward left ventricular stroke volume.

    d. Bradycardia may require prompt treatment with atropine.

6. Monitoring is dictated by the complexity of the surgery and the severity of the aortic regurgitation.

    a. A minor operation performed in a patient with asymptomatic aortic regurgitation probably does not require invasive monitoring.

    b. A pulmonary artery catheter is useful for optimizing intravascular fluid volume or when a peripheral vasodilating drug is administered in an attempt to facilitate forward left ventricular stroke volume.

VII. TRICUSPID REGURGITATION

A. Pathophysiology

1. Tricuspid regurgitation is usually functional, reflecting dilation of the right ventricle due to pulmonary hypertension. Infective endocarditis as associated with intravenous drug abuse is also a common cause of tricuspid regurgitation.

2. The basic hemodynamic consequence of tricuspid regurgitation is right atrial volume overload that is usually well tolerated.

B. Management of Anesthesia

1. A specific anesthetic drug combination or technique cannot be specifically recommended.

2. Intravascular fluid volume and central venous pressure are maintained in a high normal range to facilitate an adequate right ventricular stroke volume and left ventricular filling.

3. Central venous pressure is monitored to reflect the adequacy of intravascular fluid volume and to detect evidence of nitrous oxide-induced pulmonary vasoconstriction.

CHAPTER 3

Congenital Heart Disease

Congenital heart disease is present in about 1% of newborn infants (Table 3-1) (see Stoelting RK, Dierdorf SF. Congenital heart disease. In: Anesthesia and Co-Existing Disease. 3rd Ed. New York. Churchill Livingstone, 1993). **Signs and symptoms** of congenital heart disease manifest during the first week of life in about 50% of afflicted neonates and before 5 years of age in virtually all remaining patients (Table 3-2). **Echocardiography** is the initial diagnostic test, whereas cardiac catheterization and selective angiocardiography are the most definitive diagnostic techniques available for use in patients with congenital heart disease. Certain general problems may afflict the patient with congenital heart disease (Table 3-3). The major unresolved problem in the management of congenital heart disease is treatment of pulmonary vascular disease and associated **pulmonary hypertension**.

I. **LEFT-TO-RIGHT INTRACARDIAC SHUNT** (Table 3-1). The ultimate result of this shunt, regardless of its location, is increased pulmonary blood flow with pulmonary hypertension, right ventricular hypertrophy, and eventually congestive heart failure (CHF).

A. **Secundum atrial septal defect (ASD)** is most often located in the center of the interatrial septum.
   1. The two principal complications of an ASD are pulmonary hypertension and right ventricular hypertrophy, reflecting the chronic increase in pulmonary blood flow.
   2. **Surgical closure** of a secundum ASD is indicated when **pulmonary blood flow is at least twice systemic blood flow.** Surgery is not indicated when pulmonary hypertension is severe.

B. **Primum atrial septal defect (endocardial cushion defect)** is characterized by a large opening in the interatrial septum. Frequently it involves the mitral (mitral regurgitation) and tricuspid valves.
   1. **Treatment** is often surgical closure during the first decade of life to prevent pulmonary hypertension from becoming irreversible. Initially, palliative banding of the pulmonary artery may be selected in an attempt to reduce the magnitude of the left-to-right intracardiac shunt.

Table 3-1. *Classification and Incidence^a of Congenital Heart Disease*

Left-to-Right Intracardiac Shunt
    Secundum atrial septal defect (10%)
    Primum atrial septal defect (3%)
    Ventricular septal defect (28%)
    Patent ductus arteriosus (10%)
    Aorticopulmonary fenestration

Right-to-Left Intracardiac Shunt
    Tetralogy of Fallot (10%)
    Eisenmenger syndrome
    Ebstein's malformation of the tricuspid valve
    Tricuspid valve

Separation of the Pulmonary and Systemic Circulations
    Transposition of the great arteries (5%)

Mixing of Blood Between the Pulmonary and Systemic Circulations
    Truncus arteriosus
    Partial anomalous pulmonary venous return
    Total anomalous pulmonary venous return (1%)
    Hypoplastic left heart syndrome
    Double outlet right ventricle

Increased Myocardial Work
    Aortic stenosis (7%)
    Coarctation of the aorta (5%)
    Pulmonic stenosis (10%)

^{a} Numbers in parentheses represent approximate incidence as percentage of the total.

    2. Management of Anesthesia (Table 3-4)
  C. Ventricular septal defect (VSD) is most often an opening in the muscular ridge that separates the body of the right ventricle from the pulmonary artery outflow tract.
    1. Cardiac catheterization usually demonstrates that pulmonary blood flow exceeds systemic blood flow by 1.5 to 3 times and pulmonary vascular resistance may be moderately elevated.
    2. Treatment. When medical management is not successful, it is necessary to consider a palliative surgical procedure such as pulmonary artery banding.
    3. Management of Anesthesia (Table 3-4)

Table 3-2. *Signs and Symptoms of Congenital Heart Disease*

Infants	Children
Tachypnea	Dyspnea
Failure to gain weight	Slow physical development
Heart rate >200 beats•min^{-1}	Decreased exercise tolerance
Heart murmur	Heart murmur
Congestive heart failure	Congestive heart failure
Cyanosis	Cyanosis
	Clubbing of digits
	Squatting
	Hypertension

Table 3-3. *Common Problems Associated With Congenital Heart Disease*

Infective endocarditis (prophylactic antibiotics recommended before any dental or surgical procedure)

Cardiac dysrhythmias

Complete heart block (following surgical correction of a ventricular septal defect)

Hypertension (coarctation of the aorta and may persist after repair)

Polycythemia (response to chronic arterial hypoxemia)

Thromboembolism

Coagulopathy (defective platelet aggregation)

Brain abscess (mimics stroke)

Increased plasma uric acid concentration

a. Anesthesia for placement of a pulmonary artery band is often achieved with a drug that provides minimum cardiac depression plus a muscle relaxant to prevent patient movement.
b. If bradycardia or hypotension develops during surgery, it may be necessary to remove the pulmonary artery band promptly.
c. Third-degree atrioventricular heart block may fol-

Table 3-4. *Management of Anesthesia in the Patient With a Left-to-Right Intracardiac Shunt*

Prophylactic antibiotics

Avoid delivery of air into the circulation

Pharmacokinetics of inhaled and injected drugs unlikely to be altered

Positive-pressure ventilation well tolerated

Avoid acute and persistent increases in systemic vascular resis-tance or decreases in pulmonary vascular resistance

Transient cardiac dysrhythmias or conduction distur-bances may follow surgical repair

low surgical closure if the cardiac conduction system is near the VSD.

D. Patent ductus arteriosus (PDA) is often asymptomatic and remains unrecognized until a characteristic murmur is detected during a routine physical examination.

   1. Treatment is by surgical ligation through a left thoracotomy incision, often after the patient is >2 years of age.

   2. Management of anesthesia (Table 3-4)

   a. A volatile drug is often selected to lower blood pressure, so there is less danger of the PDA escaping from the vascular clamp or of tearing as it is being divided.

   b. Ligation of the PDA is often associated with significant systemic hypertension during the early postoperative period.

II. RIGHT-TO-LEFT INTRACARDIAC SHUNT (Table 3-1)

A. Tetralogy of Fallot is the most common congenital heart defect, producing a right-to-left intracardiac shunt with **decreased pulmonary blood flow and arterial hypoxemia.**

   1. Anatomic defects include a VSD, an aorta that overrides the pulmonary outflow tract, obstruction of the pulmonary artery outflow tract, and right ventricular hypertrophy.

   2. Signs and symptoms depend on the size of the right ventricular outflow tract (Table 3-5).

3. **Treatment** is initially with a palliative procedure designed to increase pulmonary blood flow by virtue of the anastomosis of a systemic artery to a pulmonary artery, followed at a later age by complete correction of the cardiac defect using cardiopulmonary bypass (Table 3-6).
4. **Management of anesthesia** is based on avoiding changes that would acutely increase the magnitude of the right-to-left intracardiac shunt (Table 3-7).
   a. Preoperatively, it is important to avoid dehydration by maintaining oral feedings in the very young or by providing intravenous fluids before arriving in

---

Table 3-5. *Signs and Symptoms of Tetralogy of Fallot*

Cyanosis (PaO$_2$ usually <50 mmHg)

Squatting (increases systemic vascular resistance)

Hypercyanotic attacks (sudden decrease in pulmonary blood flow often in association with exercise or crying; treatment is propranolol or phenylephrine)

Cerebrovascular accident

Cerebral abscess

Infective endocarditis

Table 3-6. *Treatment of Tetralogy of Fallot*

Initial Palliative Procedure
   Potts operation (anastomosis between the descending thoracic aorta and the left pulmonary artery)
   Waterston shunt (anastomosis between the ascending thoracic aorta and the right pulmonary artery)
   Blalock-Taussig shunt (anastomosis between a branch of the thoracic aorta and one of the pulmonary arteries)

Complete Surgical Repair
   Closure of the ventricular septal defect and enlargement of the pulmonary artery outflow tract
   Risk of third-degree atrioventricular heart block
   Platelet dysfunction

Table 3-7. *Events That Increase the Magnitude of a Right-to-Left Intracardiac Shunt*

Decreased Systemic Vascular Resistance
    Volatile anesthetics
    Histamine release
    Ganglionic blockade
    Alpha blockade

Increased Pulmonary Vascular Resistance

Increased Myocardial Contractility (may accentuate infundibular obstruction to ejection of right ventricular stroke volume)

the operating room. Crying evoked by the intramuscular administration of a drug could result in a **hypercyanotic attack.** For this reason, it may be prudent to withhold intramuscular drugs until the patient is in a highly supervised environment.

b. **Treatment of a hypercyanotic attack** is influenced by the precipitating cause (beta antagonist if due to spasm of the infundibular outflow tract and intravenous fluids and/or phenylephrine if due to decreased systemic vascular resistance).

c. **Induction of anesthesia** is often with ketamine (3 to 4 $mg \cdot kg^{-1}$ IM or 1 to 2 $mg \cdot kg^{-1}$ IV), followed by maintenance with combinations of drugs that may include ketamine, benzodiazepines, opioids, and nitrous oxide. The beneficial effect of ketamine is presumed to reflect a drug-induced increase in systemic vascular resistance that leads to a decrease in the magnitude of the right-to-left intracardiac shunt (PaO_2 often improves).

d. Intraoperative skeletal muscle paralysis is often provided by pancuronium, which maintains blood pressure and systemic vascular resistance.

e. Excessive positive airway pressure may adversely increase pulmonary vascular resistance.

f. **Intravascular fluid volume** is maintained with intravenous fluid administration, as co-existing polycythemia negates the need for early blood replacement.

g. **Phenylephrine** is useful for treating abrupt decreases in blood pressure owing to a decrease in systemic vascular resistance.

    h. Meticulous care must be taken to avoid infusion of air via tubing used to deliver intravenous solutions, as systemic air embolization might result.

B. Eisenmenger syndrome describes a situation in which the left-to-right intracardiac shunt (often through a VSD) is reversed owing to marked increases in pulmonary vascular resistance.

    1. The presence of this syndrome contraindicates surgical correction of the congenital cardiac defect.

    2. Management of anesthesia is as described for the patient with tetralogy of Fallot (Table 3-7).

C. Ebstein's malformation of the tricuspid valve is often associated with a right-to-left shunt through a patent foramen ovale or ASD. Hazards during anesthesia include the development of cardiac tachydysrhythmias (increased incidence of Wolff-Parkinson-White syndrome) and arterial hypoxemia resulting from increased magnitude of the right-to-left intracardiac shunt.

D. Tricuspid atresia is characterized by arterial hypoxemia, a small right ventricle, a large left ventricle, and markedly decreased pulmonary blood flow.

    1. Treatment is with a **Fontan procedure.** This approach involves anastomosis of the right atrial appendage to the right pulmonary artery, so as to bypass the right ventricle and provide a direct aortopulmonary communication.

    2. Management of anesthesia for the patient undergoing a Fontan procedure has been successfully achieved with opioids or volatile anesthetics.

        a. It is important to maintain an elevated right atrial pressure (16 to 20 mmHg) to facilitate pulmonary blood flow.

        b. Subsequent management of anesthesia in a patient who has undergone a Fontan procedure is facilitated by monitoring **central venous pressure (equal to pulmonary artery pressure in these patients)** for assessment of intravascular fluid volume and detection of sudden impairment of left ventricular function.

E. Foramen ovale is probe patent in about 30% of patients, such that a sudden increase in right atrial pressure can lead to a right-to-left intracardiac shunt and unexplained arterial hypoxemia or paradoxical air embolism.

III. SEPARATION OF THE PULMONARY AND SYSTEMIC CIRCULATIONS

A. **Transportation of the great arteries** is manifested as profound arterial hypoxemia at birth. Survival is not possible unless there is mixing of blood between the two circulations through an ASD, VSD, or PDA.

1. **Treatment** is an initial cardiac catheterization designed to increase pulmonary blood flow (balloon atrial septostomy; Rashkind procedure). Third-degree atrioventricular heart block may follow a balloon septostomy, necessitating prompt infusion of atropine or isoproterenol. Subsequent surgical correction using cardiopulmonary bypass is accomplished by the Mustard procedure (reversal of flow at the atrial level), the Rastelli procedure (closure of the ASD and creation of a pulmonary outflow tract with a Dacron conduit), or the Fontan procedure (see section II D1).

2. **Management of anesthesia** is often with ketamine plus pancuronium to provide skeletal muscle paralysis.

    a. Separation of the two circulations means the onset of injected drugs may be accelerated, whereas the effects of inhaled drugs may be delayed.

    b. Dehydration must be avoided, as the high hematocrit can lead to cerebral venous thrombosis.

IV. MIXING OF BLOOD BETWEEN THE PULMONARY AND SYSTEMIC CIRCULATIONS (Table 3-1)

A. **Truncus arteriosus** is present when a single arterial trunk overrides both ventricles, which are connected through a VSD.

1. **Management of anesthesia** is influenced by the magnitude of pulmonary blood flow.

    a. When pulmonary blood flow is increased, the use of positive end-expiratory pressure (PEEP) may be helpful. Increased pulmonary blood flow may be associated with evidence of myocardial ischemia on the electrocardiogram.

    b. Patients with decreased pulmonary blood flow and arterial hypoxemia should be managed as described for tetralogy of Fallot (see section II A4).

B. **Total anomalous pulmonary venous return** is character-ized by drainage of all four pulmonary veins into the sys-temic venous return in the presence of an ASD or PDA.

1. CHF is the clinical presentation in nearly every patient.

2. **Management of anesthesia** may include PEEP in an attempt to decrease excessive pulmonary blood flow or treat pulmonary edema.

a. Operative manipulation of the right atrium is often poorly tolerated.

b. Intravenous infusions may be hazardous, as an asso-ciated increase in right atrial pressure is transmit-ted directly to the pulmonary veins.

C. **Hypoplastic left heart syndrome** is characterized by left ven-tricular hypoplasia, mitral valve hypoplasia, aortic valve atre-sia, and hypoplasia of the ascending aorta.

1. Survival is dependent on the presence of a PDA and a balance between systemic vascular resistance and pul-monary vascular resistance, since both circulations are supplied from a single ventricle in a parallel fashion.

2. **Treatment** is an initial palliative procedure that elimi-nates the need for the PDA (reconstruction of the ascending aorta during whole body hypothermic circu-latory arrest), followed at a later date when the pul-monary vascular resistance has declined to adult levels by a Fontan procedure (see section II D1).

3. **Management of anesthesia** is often with an opioid plus pancuronium to provide skeletal muscle paralysis.

a. A PaO_2 >100 mmHg implies excessive pulmonary blood flow at the expense of systemic blood flow. Attempts to increase pulmonary vascular resistance (hypoventilation, PEEP) are indicated.

b. After cardiopulmonary bypass, the most frequent problem is too little pulmonary blood flow (PaO_2 <20 mmHg). Attempts to decrease pulmonary vas-cular resistance are indicated (hyperventilation, iso-proterenol).

c. A PaO_2 >50 mmHg after cardiopulmonary bypass may indicate inadequate systemic blood flow and the likelihood of progressive metabolic acidosis unless steps are taken to decrease pulmonary blood flow.

V. INCREASED MYOCARDIAL WORK (Table 3-1)

A. **Congenital aortic stenosis** (bicuspid aortic valve; may include characteristic appearance in which the facial bones are prominent) is usually asymptomatic until adulthood, when surgical replacement of the valve becomes necessary (see Chapter 2, section V).

B. **Coarctation of the Aorta**

 1. **Preductal** coarctation of the aorta is most often characterized by a localized constriction just proximal to the ductus arteriosus or by diffuse narrowing of the arch of the aorta. CHF usually is manifested during the first weeks of life.

 a. Associated cardiac defects include PDA, VSD, and bicuspid aortic valve.

 b. Surgical correction may require initial ligation of the PDA (limits blood flow to lower part of body until repair of the narrowed portion of the aorta is completed; metabolic acidosis may require treatment with sodium bicarbonate) and clamping of the left subclavian artery (monitor blood pressure by a catheter in the right radial artery).

 2. **Postductal** coarctation that manifests in a young adult characteristically involves that portion of the aorta immediately distal to the left subclavian artery. Diagnosis is often a chance finding on routine physical examination when either upper extremity hypertension (decreased blood pressure in legs and a palpable delay in the femoral pulse) or a systolic murmur is discovered.

 a. **Treatment** is with surgical resection of the stenotic portion of the aorta, when the gradient across the coarctation is >40 mmHg.

 b. **Management of anesthesia** (Table 3-8)

C. **Congenital pulmonic stenosis** is usually valvular rather than infundibular and is often associated with a probe patent foramen ovale.

 1. Arterial hypoxemia and CHF may be manifestations of severe pulmonic stenosis in neonates, whereas older patients may experience syncope, angina pectoris, and sudden death (right ventricular infarction).

 2. **Management of anesthesia** is designed to avoid an increase in right ventricular oxygen requirements as produced by an excessive increase in heart rate and myocardial contractility.

Table 3-8. *Management of Anesthesia for Correction of Coarctation of the Aorta*

Adequacy of Perfusion of the Lower Portion of the Body During Cross-clamping of the Aorta
Monitor blood pressure continuously above (right radial artery) and below (right femoral artery) the level of the coarctation
Maintain mean arterial pressure >40 mmHg in the lower extremities (kidneys, spinal cord)
Propensity for Systemic Hypertension During Cross-clamping of the Aorta
Treat with a volatile anesthetic or nitroprusside
Risk of Neurologic Sequelae Due to Ischemia of the Spinal Cord
Monitor somatosensory evoked potentials (paraplegia may still occur, as motor portion of cord is not monitored)
Postoperative Hypertension
Treat with nitroprusside with or without a beta antagonist (labetalol or hydralazine are also effective)

   a. The impact of a change in pulmonary vascular resistance (positive-pressure ventilation of the lungs) is minimized by the presence of the fixed obstruction at the pulmonic valve.

   b. It is extremely difficult to resuscitate these patients during cardiac arrest. This is because external cardiac compression is not very effective in forcing

Table 3-9. *Circulatory Anomalies That May Cause Mechanical Obstruction of the Trachea*

Double aortic arch (resulting vascular ring can produce pressure on the esophagus or trachea; place tracheal tube beyond level of compression)
Aberrant left pulmonary artery
Absent pulmonic valve (dilation of pulmonary artery may compress the trachea; intubation of trachea and continuous positive airway pressure may serve to splint the trachea)

blood across a stenotic pulmonic valve. For this reason, hypotension or cardiac dysrhythmias should be promptly treated.

VI. **MECHANICAL OBSTRUCTION OF THE TRACHEA.** The trachea may be obstructed by circulatory anomalies manifested as **unexplained stridor** or as other evidence of upper airway obstruction, particularly after placement of a nasogastric tube or an esophageal stethoscope (Table 3-9).

CHAPTER 4

Abnormalities of Cardiac Conduction and Cardiac Rhythm

Cardiac dysrhythmias that occur during the perioperative period can usually be explained on the basis of abnormalities of cardiac impulse conduction (reentry) or impulse formation (automatic or ectopic) (see Stoelting RK, Dierdorf SF. Abnormalities of cardiac conduction and cardiac rhythm. In: Anesthesia and Co-Existing Disease. 3rd Ed. New York. Churchill Livingstone, 1993). Pharmacologic or physiologic events may be responsible for initiation of reentry cardiac dysrhythmias (Table 4-1). Automatic cardiac dysrhythmias are due to enhanced automaticity (altered slope of phase 4 depolarization of the cardiac action potential) of a focus in the heart that is capable of undergoing spontaneous depolarization (repetitive firing) analogous to the sinus node (Table 4-2). The importance of cardiac dysrhythmias in the management of anesthesia relates to the effects of the specific rhythm disturbance on cardiac output and to possible interactions of antidysrhythmic drugs with those administered to produce anesthesia and skeletal muscle relaxation.

I. DIAGNOSIS

A. The electrocardiogram (ECG) is the cornerstone for the diagnosis of cardiac conduction and rhythm disturbances. **The following questions should be asked when interpreting the ECG.**

1. What is the heart rate?
2. Are P waves present? What is their relationship to the QRS complex?
3. What is the duration of the P-R interval?
4. What is the duration of the QRS complex?
5. Is the ventricular rhythm regular?
6. Are there early cardiac beats or abnormal pauses after the QRS complex?

B. **Ambulatory electrocardiographic monitoring (Holter monitoring)** is most useful in (1) documenting the occurrence of life-threatening cardiac dysrhythmias, (2) assessing the

---

Table 4-1. *Events Associated With Initiation of Cardiac Dysrhythmias During the Perioperative Period*

Arterial hypoxemia

Electrolyte disturbances
  Potassium
  Magnesium

Acid-base disturbances

Altered activity of the autonomic nervous system

Increased myocardial fiber stretch
  Hypertension
  Intubation of the trachea

Myocardial ischemia

Drugs
  Catecholamines
  Volatile anesthetics

Co-existing cardiac disease
  Pre-excitation syndrome
  Prolonged Q-T interval syndrome

---

efficacy of antidysrhythmic drug therapy, and (3) detecting the occurrence of silent (asymptomatic) myocardial ischemia.

II. TREATMENT

A. It is important to consider and correct events (PaO_2, $PaCO_2$, pH, electrolytes, autonomic nervous system activity) responsible for evoking cardiac dysrhythmias before

---

Table 4-2. *Events That Alter the Slope of Phase 4 Depolarization*

Increase Slope	Decrease Slope
Arterial hypoxemia	Vagal stimulation
Hypercarbia	Positive airway pressure
Catecholamines	Acute hyperkalemia
Sympathomimetic drugs	Hypothermia
Acute hypokalemia	
Hyperthermia	
Hypertension	

---

initiating antidysrhythmic drug therapy or placing an artificial cardiac pacemaker (Tables 4-1 and 4-2).

B. Antidysrhythmic drugs are administered when correction of identifiable precipitating events is not sufficient to suppress the cardiac dysrhythmia (Table 4-3).

1. **Lidocaine** is useful in the treatment of most ventricular cardiac dysrhythmias requiring pharmacologic treatment during the perioperative period.

   a. **Treatment of ventricular premature beats** is with a loading dose of lidocaine (1 to 2 mg·kg^{-1} IV), followed by a continuous infusion (1 to 4 mg·min^{-1} IV) to maintain a therapeutic plasma concentration of 2 to 5 μg·ml^{-1}.

   b. In the presence of decreased hepatic blood flow associated with general anesthesia, it may be necessary to decrease the lidocaine dose.

2. Drugs useful in the treatment of **atrial tachydysrhythmias** include beta antagonists, verapamil (75 to 150 μg·kg^{-1} IV over 5 minutes), digoxin, and adenosine (3 to 12 mg IV).

C. Electrical cardioversion (50 to 100 joules) is most useful in the treatment of atrial flutter, atrial fibrillation, and ventricular tachycardia (exceptions are digitalis-induced cardiac dysrhythmias, which may be enhanced by cardioversion).

1. Intravenous sedation for this treatment is provided with drugs such as methohexital, etomidate, or propofol.

2. Drugs such as atropine and lidocaine should be available (ventricular ectopy is common after treatment), as should equipment for emergency artificial cardiac pacing, in the event that underlying sinoatrial node dysfunction is manifested after successful cardioversion.

D. Artificial cardiac pacemakers inserted intravenously (endocardial lead) or by the subcostal approach (epicardial or myocardial lead) are the treatment of choice for disturbances of cardiac impulse conduction characterized as atrioventricular (AV) heart block.

1. A five-letter generic code is used to describe the various pacing modalities of artificial cardiac pacemakers (Table 4-4).

   a. The first three letters of this code describe the various types of artificial cardiac pulse generators (Table 4-5).

Table 4-3. *Cardiac Antidysrhythmic Drugs*

Agent	Indication	Side Effects
Quinidine	Atrial tachydysrhythmias Ventricular tachydysrhythmias Ventricular premature beats Atrial fibrillation Atrial flutter	Direct myocardial depression Peripheral vasodilation Hypotension Paradoxical ventricular tachycardia Thrombocytopenia Diarrhea Hepatitis Potentiates nondepo- larizing muscle relaxants
Procainamide	Ventricular tachydysrhythmias Ventricular premature beats	Direct myocardial depression Peripheral vasodilation Hypotension Paradoxical ventricular tachycardia Lupus-like syndrome Accumulation with renal dysfunction Potentiates nondepo- larizing muscle relaxants
Disopyramide	Ventricular tachydysrhythmias Atrial tachydysrhythmias	Direct myocardial depression Anticholinergic effects Paradoxical ventricular tachycardia Accumulation with renal dysfunction Potentiates nondepo- larizing muscle relaxants
Propranolol	Atrial fibrillation Atrial flutter Paroxysmal atrial tachycardia Ventricular tachydysrhythmias Digitalis-induced ventricular dysrhythmias	Sinus bradycardia Direct myocardial depression Bronchoconstriction Lethargy
Verapamil	Paroxysmal supraventricular tachycardia	Direct myocardial depression

(Continues)

Table 4-3. *Cardiac Antidysrhythmic Drugs* (Continued)

Agent	Indication	Side Effects
Verapamil (cont'd)	Atrial fibrillation Atrial flutter	Bradycardia Hypotension Potentiates depolarizing and nondepolarizing muscle relaxants Impairs antagonism of nondepolarizing neuro-muscular blockade
Digoxin	Atrial tachydysrhythmias Atrial fibrillation Atrial flutter	Toxicity, especially with renal dysfunction and/or hypokalemia
Adenosine	Paroxysmal supraventricular tachycardia (including that associated with accessory tracts)	Peripheral vasodilation Heart block
Phenytoin	Digitalis-induced supraventricular and ventricular dysrhythmias Paradoxical ventricular tachycardia	Hypotension Heart block Sedation Ataxia Hyperglycemia Gingival hyperplasia
Bretylium	Recurrent ventricular fibrillation Recurrent ventricular dysrhythmias	Initial hypertension Peripheral vasodilation Hypotension Accumulation with renal dysfunction Aggravates digitalis toxicity
Amiodarone	Supraventricular tachydysrhythmias Ventricular tachydysrhythmias	Prolonged elimination half-time Bradycardia Hypotension Pulmonary fibrosis Postoperative ventila-tory failure Skeletal muscle weakness Peripheral neuropathies Hepatitis Thyroid dysfunction Cyanotic discoloration of the face

(Continues)

Table 4-3. *Cardiac Antidysrhythmic Drugs* (Continued)

Agent	Indication	Side Effects
Amiodarone (cont'd)		Corneal deposits
Lidocaine	Ventricular premature beats Recurrent ventricular fibrillation	Accumulation with decreased hepatic blood flow Central nervous system toxicity; direct cardiac depression and peripheral vasodilation with excessive plasma concentrations

Table 4-4. *Generic Code for Identification and Description of Pacemaker Function*

First Letter	Second Letter	Third Letter	Fourth Letter	Fifth Letter
Cardiac chamber paced	Cardiac chamber in which electrical activity is sensed	Response of generator to sensed R wave and P wave	Programmable functions of the generator	Antitachycardia functions of the generator
V—Ventricle	V—Ventricle	T—Triggering	P—Programmable (rate and/or output only)	B—Bursts
A—Atrium	A—Atrium	I—Inhibited	M—Multiprogrammable	N—Normal rate competition[a]
D—Dual (atrium and ventricle)	D—Dual	D—Dual	C—Communicating[b]	S—Scanning
	O—None (asynchronous)	O—None (asynchronous)	O—None (fixed function)	E—External

[a] *Stimuli delivered at normal rates upon sensing tachycardia (underdrive pacing).*
[b] *Capability of being noninvasively interrogated.*

Table 4-5. *Types of Artificial Cardiac Pulse Generators*

Letter Number [a]			
I	II	III	**Description**
A	O	O	Asynchronous (fixed rate) atrial pacing
V	O	O	Asynchronous (fixed rate) ventricular pacing
A	A	I	Noncompetitive (demand) atrial pacing, electrical output inhibited by intrinsic atrial depolarization (P wave)
V	V	I	Noncompetitive (demand) ventricular pacing, electrical output inhibited by intrinsic ventricular depolarization (R wave)
A	A	T	Triggered atrial pacing, electrical output triggered by intrinsic atrial depolarization (P wave)
V	V	T	Triggered ventricular pacing, electrical output triggered by intrinsic ventricular depolarization (R wave)
D	V	I	Paces (sequential) in atrium and ventricle, does not sense P waves, does sense R waves
D	D	D	Paces and senses in atrium and ventricle
V	D	D	Paces in ventricle, senses in atrium and ventricle, synchronized with atrial activity and paces ventricle after a preset atrioventricular interval

[a] See Table 4-4 for definitions of letter numbers.

    b. A standard ventricular demand pacemaker is classified as VVI, whereas an AV pacemaker with two pacing electrodes is classified as DVI (preservation of the atrial and ventricular contraction is described as physiologic pacing).

    c. Early pacemaker failure is usually due to electrode displacement or breakage, whereas failures >6 months after implantation are most often due to premature battery depletion or to a faulty pulse generator.

    d. Improved shielding of artificial cardiac pacemakers has largely eliminated problems of pacemaker inhibition due to extraneous electrical fields (microwaves, electrocautery, magnetic resonance imaging).

    e. A demand pacemaker may be overridden by the intrinsic heart rate if this rate is more rapid. Also, the pacemaker can be momentarily converted to an asynchronous mode by placing a magnet externally over the pulse generator.

2. **Noninvasive transcutaneous cardiac pacing** is an alternative to emergency transvenous artificial cardiac pacemaker placement.

3. **Preoperative evaluation** of the patient with an artificial cardiac pacemaker includes determination of the reason for placing the pacemaker and an assessment of its present function.

   a. A preoperative history of vertigo or syncope or a 10% decrease in the discharge rate of an asynchronous cardiac pacemaker (usually 70 to 72 beats·min^{-1}) may reflect pacemaker dysfunction.

   b. The ECG is evaluated to confirm 1:1 capture, as evidenced by a pacemaker spike for every palpated peripheral pulse. (This is not helpful, however, in the patient with an intrinsic heart rate greater than the artificial cardiac pacemaker rate.)

   c. Proper function of a demand pacemaker can be confirmed by demonstrating the appearance of captured beats on the ECG when the pacemaker is converted to the asynchronous mode by placement of an **external converter magnet** over the pulse generator.

   d. A chest radiograph is useful to confirm the absence of a break in the pacemaker electrodes.

4. **Management of anesthesia** in the patient with an artificial cardiac pacemaker includes monitoring to confirm continued function of the pulse generator and ready availability of equipment and drugs to maintain an acceptable intrinsic heart rate should the artificial cardiac pacemaker unexpectedly fail (Table 4-6).

   a. There is no evidence that anesthetics or events associated with the perioperative period alter the stimu-

---

Table 4-6. *Management of Anesthesia in the Patient With an Artificial Cardiac Pacemaker*

Continuous monitoring of the electrocardiogram
Continuous monitoring of a peripheral pulse
Electrical defibrillator present
External converter magnet available
Drugs prepared—atropine, isoproterenol

lation threshold of an artificial cardiac pacemaker.

b. Skeletal muscle myopotentials (fasciculations) produced by succinylcholine may inhibit a normal-functioning artificial cardiac pacemaker by causing contraction of skeletal muscle groups (myopotential inhibition) interpreted as intrinsic R waves by the pulse generator. Nevertheless, clinical experience suggests that succinylcholine is generally a safe drug.

c. Despite improved shielding of the artificial cardiac pacemaker, it is still a reasonable recommendation to place the **ground plate for the electrocautery** as far as possible from the pulse generator. This step minimizes detection of the current by the pulse generator.

5. Anesthesia for Pacemaker Insertion

a. A functioning transvenous artificial cardiac pacemaker should be in place or a noninvasive transcutaneous cardiac pacemaker available before induction of anesthesia for permanent artificial cardiac pacemaker placement.

b. The presence of a transvenous pacemaker predisposes the patient to the risk of ventricular fibrillation from microshock levels of electrical current.

III. DISTURBANCES OF CARDIAC IMPULSE CONDUCTION. Heart block that occurs above the AV node is usually benign and transient, whereas heart block that develops below the AV node tends to be both progressive and permanent (Table 4-7).

IV. DISTURBANCES OF CARDIAC RHYTHM. Cardiac dysrhythmias that arise in the atria or AV node are defined as supraventricular dysrhythmias, whereas those that arise below the AV node are defined as ventricular dysrhythmias (Table 4-8).

V. PRE-EXCITATION SYNDROMES

A. These syndromes reflect the presence of a congenital accessory (anomalous) pathway that bypasses the AV node. These pathways are present in 0.1% to 0.3% of the population, most often manifesting as **paroxysmal supraventricular tachycardia** that may result in syncope and/or congestive heart failure (Table 4-9).

Table 4-7. *Classification of Heart Block*

First-Degree AV Heart Block
  P-R interval >0.2 second
  Usually asymptomatic
  Atropine effective
Second-Degree AV Heart Block
  Mobitz type 1 (progressive prolongation of P-R
    interval until a beat is entirely blocked)
  Mobitz type 2 (sudden interruption of cardiac con-
    duction; frequently progressive to third-degree
    AV heart block)
Unifascicular Heart Block
Right Bundle Branch Block
  QRS >0.1 second
  Usually benign
Left Bundle Branch Block
  QRS >0.12 second and wide notched R waves in
    all leads
  Often associated with ischemic heart disease
Bifascicular Heart Block
  No evidence that risk of third-degree AV heart
    block is increased during surgery
Third-Degree AV Heart Block
  Heart rate depends on site of block (near AV node
    45–55 beats·min^{-1}; below AV node 30–40
    beats·min^{-1} and QRS complexes wide)
  Isoproterenol (1–4 μg·min^{-1} IV) plus atropine is a
    chemical pacemaker
  Permanent artificial cardiac pacemaker

Table 4-8. *Disturbances of Cardiac Rhythm*

Supraventricular Dysrhythmias
  Sinus tachycardia (>120 beats·min^{-1}; anxiety, pain,
    sepsis, hypovolemia, hypoxemia, hypoglycemia,
    light anesthesia)
  Sinus bradycardia (<60 beats·min^{-1}; athlete, beta
    antagonists, vagal stimulation, hypothermia)
  Sick sinus syndrome (bradycardia punctuated by
    tachycardia; treatment: artificial cardiac pacemaker)

(Continues)

Table 4-8. *Disturbances of Cardiac Rhythm* (Continued)

Supraventricular Dysrhythmias *(cont'd)*
  Atrial and junctional premature beats (early and abnormally shaped P waves; treatment: atropine)
  Paroxysmal supraventricular tachycardia (treatment: vagal maneuvers, beta antagonists, verapamil, adenosine, electrical cardioversion)
  Atrial flutter
  Atrial fibrillation (initial treatment: often digoxin)
  Junctional (nodal) rhythm (initial treatment: atropine)
  Wandering atrial pacemaker
Ventricular Dysrhythmias
  Ventricular premature beats (arterial hypoxemia, myocardial ischemia, sympathetic nervous system activation; treatment: removal of cause and administration of lidocaine)
  Ventricular tachycardia (treatment: lidocaine if hemodynamically tolerated, otherwise electrical cardioversion)
  Ventricular fibrillation (prompt institution of electrical defibrillation; lidocaine or bretylium may improve response)

Table 4-9. *Pathophysiology of Pre-excitation Syndromes*

Nomenclature	Accessory Pathway Connections	Electrocardiographic Manifestations
Kent's bundle (accessory atrioventricular pathway; Wolff-Parkinson-White syndrome)	Atrium to ventricle	Short P-R interval (<0.12 sec) Wide QRS complex (>0.12 sec) Delta wave
James fibers (intranodal bypass tract; Lown-Ganong-Levine syndrome)	Intranodal bypass	Short P-R interval Normal QRS complex No delta wave
Mahaim fiber (nodoventricular or fasciculoventricular pathway)	Atrioventricular node to ventricle His bundle or bundle branch to ventricle	Normal to short P-R interval Wide QRS complex Delta wave

B. **Wolff-Parkinson-White (WPW) syndrome** is the most common of the pre-excitation syndromes. The first evidence of WPW syndrome may be during the perioperative period.

1. **Treatment** of WPW syndrome is determined by the type of supraventricular dysrhythmia manifested (Table 4-10). Options available when medical management is not effective include antidysrhythmia surgery (division or cryoablation of accessory pathways) or catheter ablation (radiofrequency) techniques as guided by electrophysiologic mapping studies.

2. **Management of anesthesia** is designed to avoid any event (increased sympathetic nervous system activity, hypovolemia) or drug (digoxin) that would enhance conduction of the cardiac impulse through the accessory pathways.

   a. Concentrations of a volatile anesthetic sufficient to prevent sympathetic nervous system responses produced by intense stimulation are recommended.

   b. Pancuronium or ketamine are unlikely drug selections.

   c. Drug-enhanced antagonism of nondepolarizing muscle relaxants is acceptable.

   d. Electrical cardioversion and drugs known to be effective in the management of acute atrial tachydysrhythmias should be promptly available (Table 4-10).

Table 4-10. *Treatment of Cardiac Dysrhythmias in the Patient With Wolff-Parkinson-White Syndrome*

Paroxysmal Supraventricular Tachycardia
  Vagal maneuvers
    Valsalva
    Gag reflex (finger in the throat)
    Immersion of face in cold water (diving reflex)
  Adenosine 3–12 mg IV
  Verapamil 2.5–10 mg IV
  Esmolol 50–100 mg IV
  Procainamide 500 mg IV
  Artificial cardiac (overdrive) pacing (transvenous)
  Electrical cardioversion

Atrial Fibrillation
  Electrical cardioversion (hemodynamically unstable)
  Esmolol (hemodynamically stable)
  Procainamide (hemodynamically stable)

VI. PROLONGED Q-T INTERVAL SYNDROME (Table 4-11)

A. The diagnostic feature is a prolonged Q-T interval (>0.44 second) on the ECG.

    1. Syncope associated with this syndrome may be confused with a seizure disorder if an ECG is not obtained.

    2. An ECG to rule out prolonged Q-T interval syndrome is useful in a child with congenital deafness or with a family history of sudden death.

B. Treatment is empirical based on the presumption that the prolonged Q-T interval syndrome is due to **asymmetric sympathetic nervous system innervation of the heart** (increased left cardiac sympathetic nervous system activity or decreased right cardiac sympathetic nerve activity) (Table 4-12).

C. Management of Anesthesia

    1. General anesthesia may trigger a life-threatening ventricular dysrhythmia and cardiac arrest in the patient with prolonged Q-T interval syndrome. For this reason, consideration may be given to establishing beta-blockade or performance of a prophylactic left stellate ganglion block before induction of anesthesia.

Table 4-11. *Prolonged Q-T Interval Syndrome*

> Congenital
>   Jervell and Lange-Nielson syndrome (deafness present)
>   Romano-Ward syndrome (deafness absent)
> Acquired
>   Quinidine
>   Disopyramide
>   Tricyclic antidepressants
>   Subarachnoid hemorrhage
>   Hypokalemia
>   Hypomagnesemia
>   Right radical neck dissection

Table 4-12. *Treatment of the Prolonged Q-T Interval Syndrome*

> Beta antagonist therapy
> Left stellate ganglion block
> Left stellate ganglionectomy

2. Events known to prolong the Q-T interval (abrupt increases in sympathetic nervous system activity, acute hypokalemia) are avoided.

   a. Pharmacologic preoperative medication is provided to decrease anxiety.

   b. Intubation of the trachea is attempted only after establishing a depth of anesthesia deemed sufficient to blunt the effects of noxious stimulation.

   c. The choice of volatile anesthetic is influenced not only by its ability to suppress sympathetic nervous system responses to painful stimulation, but also to avoid sensitization of the heart to the arrhythmogenic effects of catecholamines.

   d. Drug-enhanced reversal of nondepolarizing muscle relaxants does not seem to alter the Q-T interval adversely.

   e. A beta antagonist is useful for the treatment of an acute ventricular dysrhythmia that develops intraoperatively.

CHAPTER 5

Hypertension

Hypertension is the most common circulatory derangement, affecting an estimated 60 million Americans (see Stoelting RK, Dierdorf SF. Hypertension. In: Anesthesia and Co-Existing Disease. 3rd Ed. New York. Churchill Livingstone, 1993). **Essential (primary) hypertension** accounts for more than 90% of afflicted patients and has no identifiable cause, whereas **secondary hypertension** has a demonstrable etiology (most often renal disease) (Table 5-1). The definition of hypertension is arbitrary, but it is generally agreed that a systolic blood pressure >160 mmHg and/or a diastolic blood pressure >90 mmHg constitutes hypertension, regardless of age. Hypertension is a significant risk factor for the development of ischemic heart disease and a major cause of congestive heart failure (CHF), renal failure, and cerebrovascular accident (stroke) (Fig. 5-1).

I. TREATMENT (Table 5-2)

    A. Initial drug therapy of hypertension may be with a diuretic, angiotensin-converting enzyme (ACE) inhibitor, or beta antagonist.

        1. ACE inhibitors are associated with minimal side effects (hyperkalemia is possible in patients with renal insufficiency) and high patient compliance.

        2. Single-drug therapy with a beta antagonist appears to be most effective in the patient <40 years of age.

    B. Combination drug therapy is based on the observation that efficacy of a single drug is often offset by homeostatic (baroreceptor-mediated) compensation.

II. MANAGEMENT OF ANESTHESIA (Table 5-3)

    A. Drugs showing efficacy in controlling blood pressure in an individual patient should be continued throughout the perioperative period, to ensure optimum medical control of blood pressure.

    B. Preoperative Evaluation

        1. The adequacy of blood pressure control is determined. Ideally, hypertensive patients are rendered normotensive before performance of elective surgery. There is no evidence, however, that the incidence of postopera-

Table 5-1. *Causes of Secondary Hypertension*

Etiology	Screening Test
Renal disease (pyelonephritis, glomerulonephritis, diabetic nephropathy, vascular disease)	Pyelogram Renin activity Angiography
Coarctation	Chest radiograph
Hyperadrenocorticism (Cushing's disease)	Plasma cortisol after dexamethasone suppression
Pheochromocytoma	Urine metanephrine or vanillyl-mandelic acid Clonidine suppression test Plasma catecholamines
Primary aldosteronism	Plasma and urine potassium
Drugs	Drug screen
Intracranial hypertension	

tive cardiac complications is increased when a hypertensive patient undergoes an elective operation, as long as the preoperative diastolic blood pressure is <110 mmHg (Table 5-4).

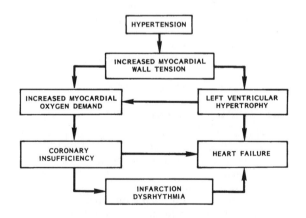

Fig. 5-1. *Chronic increases in systemic blood pressure initiate a series of pathophysiologic changes that may culminate in congestive heart failure.*

Table 5-2. *Drugs Used in the Treatment of Hypertension*

Diuretics
  Thiazides
  Potassium-sparing diuretics
  Combination of thiazide and
    potassium-sparing diuretic
  Loop diuretic

Angiotensin-Converting Enzyme Inhibitors
  Captopril
  Enalapril
  Lisinopril

Calcium Entry Blockers
  Diltiazem
  Nifedipine
  Verapamil

Vasodilators
  Hydralazine
  Minoxidil

Sympatholytics
  Beta antagonists
  Combined alpha and beta antagonist
    Labetalol
  Clonidine
  Guanabenz
  Methyldopa
  Guanadrel
  Prazosin

Table 5-3. *Management of Anesthesia for the Hypertensive Patient*

Preoperative Evaluation
  Determine adequacy of blood pressure control
  Review pharmacology of antihypertensive drugs
  Detect associated organ dysfunction
    Orthostatic hypotension
    Ischemic heart disease
    Cerebrovascular disease
    Peripheral vascular disease
    Renal dysfunction

(Continues)

Table 5-3. *Management of Anesthesia for the Hypertensive Patient* (Continued)

Induction of Anesthesia
Expect exaggerated blood pressure changes
Perform short-duration laryngoscopy

Maintenance of Anesthesia
Administer volatile anesthetic to control blood pressure
Monitor for myocardial ischemia

Postoperative Management
Anticipate hypertension
Maintain intraoperative monitoring

Table 5-4. *Risk of General Anesthesia and Elective Surgery in the Hypertensive Patient*

Blood Pressure Status Before Operation	Incidence of Perioperative Hypertensive Episodes (%)	Incidence of Postoperative Cardiac Complications (%)
Normotensive	8[a]	11
Treated and rendered normotensive	27	24
Treated but remain hypertensive	25	7
Untreated and hypertensive	20	12

[a] $P<0.5$, compared with other groups in same column.
(Data from Goldman L, Caldera DL. Risk of general anesthesia and elective operation in the hypertensive patient. Anesthesiology 1979;50:285–92.)

2. It is important to review the pharmacology and potential side effects of the drugs being used to treat hypertension (Table 5-5).
3. The presence of associated organ dysfunction (endorgan damage) is evaluated preoperatively (Table 5-6).

C. Induction of Anesthesia
   1. An exaggerated decrease in blood pressure is likely, particularly if hypertension is present preoperatively.

Table 5-5. *Potential Side Effects of Antihypertensive Drugs*

Thiazide Diuretics

Hypokalemia	Hyperglycemia
Hypomagnesemia	Hypercholesterolemia
Hyperuricemia	Decreased lithium clearance
Hypercalcemia	Dermatitis
Alkalosis	Photosensitivity

Potassium-Sparing Diuretics

Hyperkalemia
Hyponatremia
Megaloblastic anemia
Dermatitis

Angiotensin-Converting Enzyme Inhibitors

Hyperkalemia	Fetal death
Proteinuria	Dermatitis
Cough	Angioedema

Beta Antagonists

Congestive heart failure	Raynaud's phenomenon
Bradycardia	Sedation
Bronchospasm	Angina with abrupt discontinuation
Masking of hypoglycemia	Paresthesias

Calcium Entry Blockers

Bradycardia	Weakness
Tachycardia	Hepatic dysfunction
Heart block	Syncope
Congestive heart failure	

Clonidine

Sedation	Heart block
Orthostatic hypotension	Dry mouth
Rebound hypertension	Impaired glucose tolerance
Bradycardia	

Methyldopa

Sedation	Positive Coombs test
Orthostatic hypotension	Exacerbation of parkinsonism
Rebound hypertension	
Hepatotoxicity	

Prazosin

Sedation	Orthostatic hypotension
Weakness	Tachycardia

(Continues)

Table 5-5. *Potential Side Effects of Antihypertensive Drugs* (Continued)

Hydralazine

Tachycardia
Lupus-like syndrome
Fever

Minoxidil

Orthostatic hypotension	Sodium and water retention
Tachycardia	Hemodilution
Congestive heart failure	Pericardial effusion
Hypertrichosis	Nonspecific T wave changes

Table 5-6. *Preoperative Evaluation of Associated Organ Damage*

Kidneys
    Blood urea nitrogen/creatinine
    Electrolytes

Heart
    Electrocardiogram (cardiomegaly, ischemia)

Brain
    Dizziness/syncope

Peripheral Vascular Disease
    Claudication

      Ketamine is an unlikely selection, whereas other intravenous drugs are acceptable.

2. Direct laryngoscopy and intubation of the trachea may result in exaggerated increases in blood pressure, even if the patient has been rendered normotensive before surgery. Attenuation of the circulatory response during laryngoscopy is a consideration (Table 5-7).

3. Evidence of myocardial ischemia on the electrocardiogram of a patient with ischemic heart disease is most likely to occur in association with increases in blood pressure and heart rate that accompany the intubation sequence.

D. Maintenance of Anesthesia

1. The goal during maintenance of anesthesia is to adjust the depth of anesthesia in an appropriate direction (volatile anesthetics can be useful), to minimize wide

---

Table 5-7. *Methods to Attenuate Circulatory Response to Laryngoscopy*

Establish surgical level of anesthesia with a volatile anesthetic

Short-acting opioid (fentanyl 50–150 µg IV) before initiating laryngoscopy

Brief duration (<15 sec) of direct laryngoscopy

Supplemental therapy
 Laryngotracheal lidocaine
 Intravenous lidocaine
 Esmolol
 Nitroprusside

---

fluctuations in blood pressure. **Management of intraoperative blood pressure lability with the anesthetic technique may be more important than preoperative control of hypertension.**

 a. The most likely intraoperative change in blood pressure is hypertension produced by painful stimulation.

 b. A volatile anesthetic is useful for attenuating activity of the sympathetic nervous system, which is responsible for the pressor response (see Fig. 1-2).

 c. Hypotension is treated by decreasing the delivered concentration of volatile anesthetic and increasing the rate of intravenous fluid administration. A sympathomimetic drug (ephedrine, phenylephrine) may be necessary to restore vital organ perfusion pressure, until the underlying cause of hypotension can be corrected.

 d. Selection of monitors is influenced by the complexity of the surgery. Invasive monitoring is useful when emergency surgery is required in the presence of uncontrolled hypertension.

 2. Regional anesthesia is an acceptable selection for the hypertensive patient, recognizing that a need for high sensory levels of anesthesia and associated sympathetic nervous system denervation could unmask unsuspected hypovolemia.

E. Postoperative Management

 1. Hypertension during the early postoperative period is

Table 5-8. *Causes of a Hypertensive Crisis*

Chronic essential hypertension

Renovascular hypertension

Sudden withdrawal from antihypertensive therapy (central acting and beta antagonists)

Drug ingestion (cocaine, LSD, amphetamine, tricyclic antidepressants)

Pregnancy-induced hypertension (eclampsia)

Head injury

Pheochromocytoma

Guillain-Barré syndrome

Spinal cord injury

Collagen vascular diseases

Thoracic aorta dissection

not an unexpected response in the patient with preoperative hypertension.

2. The development of postoperative hypertension warrants prompt assessment (pain, fluid overload) and treatment (opioids, hydralazine, nitroprusside, labetalol) to decrease the risks of myocardial ischemia, cardiac dysrhythmias, CHF, stroke, and bleeding.

III. HYPERTENSIVE CRISIS

A. A hypertensive crisis is arbitrarily defined as a sudden increase of the diastolic blood pressure to >130 mmHg (encephalopathy, CHF, and oliguria may be present).

B. Causes of a hypertensive crisis are multiple (Table 5-8).

C. Treatment is with intravenous administration of nitroprusside during continuous monitoring of intra-arterial blood pressure and urine output.

CHAPTER 6

Congestive Heart Failure

Congestive heart failure (CHF) is most often due to (1) cardiac valve abnormalities, (2) impaired myocardial contractility secondary to ischemic heart disease or cardiomyopathy, (3) systemic hypertension, or (4) pulmonary hypertension (cor pulmonale) (see Stoelting RK, Dierdorf SF. Congestive heart failure. In: Anesthesia and Co-Existing Disease. 3rd Ed. New York. Churchill Livingstone, 1993). The presence of CHF during the preoperative period is the most important single abnormality shown to contribute to postoperative cardiac morbidity and mortality.

I. ADAPTIVE PHYSIOLOGIC MECHANISMS (Table 6-1)

II. HEMODYNAMIC PARAMETERS OF VENTRICULAR FUNCTION

A. **Cardiac function** is decreased (<2.5 L$\cdot$min$^{-1}\cdot$m^{-2}) in the presence of severe CHF.

B. **Ejection fraction** is decreased (<0.56) in the presence of decreased myocardial contractility.

C. **End-diastolic pressure** that parallels end-diastolic volume is increased in the presence of CHF. Left ventricular end-diastolic pressure is normally <12 mmHg, whereas right ventricular end-diastolic pressure is normally <5 mmHg.

III. MANIFESTATIONS OF LEFT VENTRICULAR FAILURE (Table 6-2)

IV. MANIFESTATIONS OF RIGHT VENTRICULAR FAILURE (Table 6-3)

V. TREATMENT OF CONGESTIVE HEART FAILURE

A. When symptoms persist despite correction of reversible causes, the three cornerstones of the pharmacologic treatment of CHF are digitalis, diuretics, and vasodilators.

B. Digitalis is the only orally effective positive inotropic drug in common use. Several preparations of digitalis are available, but a detailed knowledge of digoxin is sufficient for most situations (Table 6-4).

Table 6-1. *Adaptive Mechanisms That Allow the Heart to Maintain Its Cardiac Output*

Frank-Starling relation (increase in stroke volume that accompanies an increase in end-diastolic pressure)

Inotropic state (reflected by maximum velocity of contraction, V_{max})

Afterload

Heart rate

Myocardial hypertrophy and dilation

Sympathetic nervous system activity

Humoral-mediated responses

Table 6-2. *Manifestations of Left Ventricular Failure*

Fatigue

Dyspnea (interstitial pulmonary edema)

Orthopnea

Paroxysmal nocturnal dyspnea

Acute pulmonary edema (treat with morphine 5–10 mg IV, furosemide 10–40 mg IV, dopamine, digoxin; radiographic changes may persist for 1–4 days after normalization of cardiac filling pressures)

Tachypnea and rales

Tachycardia and peripheral vasoconstriction

Oliguria

Pleural effusion

Table 6-3. *Manifestations of Right Ventricular Failure*

Systemic venous congestion (jugular venous distension; also present with constrictive pericarditis or cardiac tamponade)

Hepatomegaly

Ascites

Peripheral edema (dependent and pitting)

Table 6-4. *Characteristics of Frequently Used Digitalis Preparations*

	Digoxin	Ouabain	Digitoxin
Absorption from the gastrointestinal tract	Good	Erratic	Excellent
Onset of action after intravenous administration (min)	15–30	5–10	30–120
Peak effect (h)	1.5–5	0.5–2	4–12
Elimination half-time (h)	31–33	21	120–168
Principal route of elimination	Kidneys	Kidneys	Hepatic
Average digitalizing dose (mg)			
Intravenous	0.75–1.0	0.3–0.5	0.7–1.0
Oral (during 12–24 h)	0.75–1.5		0.7–1.2
Average daily maintenance dose (adults with normal liver and renal function)			
Oral (mg)	0.125–0.5		0.05–0.2
Therapeutic plasma concentration (ng•ml^{-1})	1–1.5	0.5	15–25

1. Digoxin is excreted principally by the kidneys (parallels creatinine clearance).
2. Sensitivity to digoxin can be increased during the perioperative period if there are associated decreases in renal function or development of hypokalemia.
3. **Prophylactic use of digitalis** is controversial in the patient undergoing elective surgery without evidence of CHF. Elderly patients undergoing thoracic surgery may benefit. There are no data to support discontinuing digitalis preoperatively, especially if the drug is being administered to control heart rate.
4. **Digitalis toxicity** should be suspected during the preoperative period if (1) the patient complains of nausea and vomiting, (2) there is evidence of cardiac dysrhythmias and/or heart block on the electrocardiogram, and (3) the plasma concentration of digoxin is >3 ng•ml^{-1}.
   a. **Treatment** of digitalis toxicity includes correction of predisposing events (especially hypokalemia),

pharmacologic treatment of cardiac dysrhythmias (lidocaine, phenytoin), and insertion of a temporary transvenous cardiac pacemaker if complete heart block is present.

  b. **Surgery in the Presence of Digitalis Toxicity.** When surgery cannot be delayed, it is important to avoid (1) drugs that stimulate the sympathetic nervous system (ketamine), and (2) hyperventilation of the lungs. Volatile anesthetics may be useful selections in the presence of digitalis toxicity.

C. Diuretics

  1. The plasma potassium concentration should be determined periodically when thiazide diuretics are administered chronically, especially if the patient is also to be treated with a digitalis preparation.

  2. Chronic oral administration of loop diuretics can result in hypovolemia, orthostatic hypotension, and hypokalemia.

D. Vasodilators

  1. The present trend in the pharmacologic treatment of CHF is to optimize cardiac output by manipulating the peripheral circulation with vasodilators (Table 6-5).

  2. Vasodilators increase cardiac output by decreasing impedance to the forward ejection of left ventricular stroke volume.

Table 6-5. *Vasodilator Drugs Used in Therapy for Congestive Heart Failure*

	Effect on Venous System	Effect on Arterial System	Peak Action (h)	Duration of Effect (h)	Usual Dose and Route
Nitroglycerin	+++	+			$0.5–5\ \mu g \cdot kg^{-1} \cdot min^{-1}$ IV
Hydralazine	0	+++	1–2	4–6	25–100 mg PO
Nitroprusside	+++	+++			$0.5–5\ \mu g \cdot kg^{-1} \cdot min^{-1}$ IV
Prazosin	++	++	1–2	4–6	1–5 mg PO
Captopril	++	+++	1–2	4–8	25–75 mg PO
Enalapril	++	+++	4–8	18–30	5–40 mg PO
Lisinopril	++	+++	2–6	18–30	5–40 mg PO

    a. The limiting factor in the treatment of CHF with vasodilators is hypotension.

    b. Invasive monitoring (arterial and pulmonary artery catheter) is useful for determining changes in cardiac filling pressures and cardiac output and for calculating systemic and pulmonary vascular resistance.

E. Beta Agonists

  1. Intravenous infusions of dopamine and/or dobutamine are commonly used during the perioperative period in an effort to improve myocardial contractility. Combinations of dopamine and dobutamine provide the desirable renal effects of dopamine and the beta effects of dobutamine at doses unlikely to increase afterload, by virtue of alpha receptor stimulation.

  2. It is useful to monitor the effects of beta agonists on cardiac output and cardiac filling pressures using a pulmonary artery catheter.

VI. SURGERY IN THE PRESENCE OF CONGESTIVE HEART FAILURE

A. If surgery cannot be deferred, drugs and techniques chosen to provide anesthesia in the presence of CHF are often selected with the goal of optimizing cardiac output.

B. General Anesthesia

  1. Ketamine is a useful drug for induction of anesthesia in the presence of CHF.

  2. Administration of a volatile anesthetic must be performed cautiously, in view of the dose-dependent cardiac depressant effects produced by these drugs.

  3. In the presence of severe CHF, the use of an opioid as the only drug for maintenance of anesthesia may be justified.

  4. Positive-pressure ventilation of the lungs may be beneficial by decreasing pulmonary congestion and improving arterial oxygenation.

  5. Invasive monitoring of arterial pressure as well as cardiac filling pressures is justified when major operations are necessary in the presence of CHF.

  6. Support of cardiac output with drugs such as dopamine or dobutamine may be necessary.

  7. Drug interactions in patients treated with digitalis

should be anticipated (pancuronium, calcium), while avoiding hyperventilation of the lungs.

C. **Regional anesthesia** is an acceptable selection to provide anesthesia for a peripheral operation in the presence of CHF.

CHAPTER 7

Cardiomyopathies

Cardiomyopathies are attributable to many diverse causes but have in common **progressive and life-threatening congestive heart failure (CHF)** (Table 7-1) (see Stoelting RK, Dierdorf SF. Cardiomyopathies. In: Anesthesia and Co-Existing Disease. 3rd Ed. New York. Churchill Livingstone, 1993). Cardiomyopathies may be classified on a morphologic and hemodynamic basis as (1) dilated, (2) hypertrophic, (3) restrictive, and (4) obliterative (Table 7-2).

I. DILATED CARDIOMYOPATHY

A. **Myocardial contractility** is reduced, manifesting as decreased cardiac output and increased ventricular filling pressure. Ventricular dilation may be so marked that functional mitral and/or tricuspid regurgitation occurs. Cardiac dysrhythmias (ventricular premature beats and atrial fibrillation) are common, and the ejection fraction is <0.4. Systemic embolization is common, reflecting formation of mural thrombi in dilated and hypokinetic cardiac chambers.

B. **Multiple myocardial infarctions** produced by diffuse coronary artery disease are the most common cause of dilated cardiomyopathy.

C. There is a striking association between **alcohol abuse** and dilated cardiomyopathy.

D. The most common complication is progressive and often fatal CHF. **Sudden death** caused by cardiac dysrhythmias is frequent, as is evidence of systemic and/or pulmonary embolism.

E. **Treatment** invokes principles for management of CHF (see Chapter 6), anticoagulation if systemic embolism is a threat, and occasionally revascularization surgery or cardiac transplantation.

F. **Management of Anesthesia**
1. Goals include avoidance of drug-induced myocardial depression, maintenance of normovolemia, and prevention of increases in ventricular afterload.
a. Excessive cardiovascular depression in response to induction of anesthesia in a patient with a history of alcohol abuse may reflect unsuspected dilated cardiomyopathy.

Table 7-1. *Etiology of Cardiomyopathies*

Infectious	Viral
	Bacterial
Toxic	Alcohol
	Daunorubicin
	Doxorubicin
	Cocaine
Systemic	Muscular dystrophy
	Myotonic dystrophy
	Collagen vascular diseases
	Sarcoidosis
	Pheochromocytoma
	Acromegaly
	Thyrotoxicosis
	Myxedema
Infiltrative	Amyloidosis
	Hemochromatosis
	Primary or metastatic tumors
Nutritional	
Ischemic	
Idiopathic	

    b. Dose-dependent direct myocardial depression produced by volatile anesthetics must be considered, although the vasodilating properties of isoflurane would theoretically be desirable.

    c. Opioids are associated with benign effects on cardiac contractility. However, when used alone, they may not produce an unconscious state. An opioid administered with nitrous oxide or a benzodiazepine may result in unexpected depression of myocardial contractility.

    d. A pulmonary artery catheter is useful for guiding volume replacement and early recognition of the need for inotropic support or administration of peripheral vasodilating drugs.

  2. Regional anesthesia may be an alternative to general anesthesia in selected patients with dilated cardiomyopathy.

Table 7-2. *Classification of Cardiomyopathies on Morphologic and Hemodynamic Basis*

Factors	Type of Cardiomyopathy			
	Dilated	**Restrictive**	**Hypertrophic**	**Obliterative**
Morphology	Biventricu-lar dilation	Decreased ventricular compliance	Hypertrophy of left ventricle and usually interventricular septum	Thickened endocardium or mural thrombi
Ventricular volume	↑↑	Normal or ↑	Normal or ↓	↓
Ejection fraction	↓↓	Normal or ↓	↑↑	Normal or ↓
Ventricular compliance	Normal or ↓	↓↓	↓↓	↓↓
Ventricular filling pressure	↑↑	↑↑	Normal or ↑	↑
Stroke volume	↓↓	Normal or ↓	Normal or ↑	Normal or ↓

II. RESTRICTIVE CARDIOMYOPATHY

   A. Impaired diastolic filling produces a clinical and hemodynamic picture (increased filling pressures and decreased cardiac output) that mimics constrictive pericarditis (see Chapter 9).

   B. There is no effective treatment for restrictive cardiomyopathy. Death is usually due to cardiac dysrhythmias or intractable CHF.

   C. Management of anesthesia invokes the same principles outlined for patients with cardiac tamponade (see Chapter 9).

III. HYPERTROPHIC CARDIOMYOPATHY

   A. There is often evidence of hereditary transmission. The basic genetic defect is in the contractile elements of the heart (increased density of calcium channels), manifesting as unexplained myocardial hypertrophy.

1. In its severest form, the left ventricular chamber becomes elongated and slit-like.
2. Even in the presence of severe left ventricular outflow obstruction, the ejection fraction is >0.8, reflecting the hypercontractile condition of the heart.
3. The degree of left ventricular outflow obstruction is influenced by myocardial contractility, preload, and afterload (Table 7-3).

B. It is generally agreed that known afflicted patients should not participate in competitive sports because of the risk of sudden death (presumably due to acute left ventricular outflow obstruction or cardiac dysrhythmias).

C. **Clinical Features** (Table 7-4)

D. **Treatment** is directed at relieving the obstruction to left ventricular outflow, which may be fixed or dynamic (Table 7-3).
   1. Nitroglycerin should not be administered to the patient with hypertrophic cardiomyopathy and angina pectoris.
   2. Surgical myotomy or myomectomy of the left ventricular outflow tract is usually reserved for symptomatic patients with outflow gradients >50 mmHg.

Table 7-3. *Factors That Influence Left Ventricular Outflow Obstruction in Patients With Hypertrophic Cardiomyopathy*

Events That Increase Outflow Obstruction	Events That Decrease Outflow Obstruction
Increased myocardial contractility	Decreased myocardial contractility
Beta stimulation	Beta blockade (propra-
(catecholamines)	nolol, esmolol)
Digitalis	Volatile anesthetics
Tachycardia	(halothane)
	Calcium entry blockers
Decreased preload	
Hypovolemia	Increased preload
Vasodilators (nitroglycerin,	Hypervolemia
nitroprusside)	Bradycardia
Tachycardia	
Positive-pressure ventilation	Increased afterload
	Alpha stimulation
Decreased afterload	(phenylephrine)
Hypotension	Hypervolemia
Hypovolemia	
Vasodilators	

Table 7-4. *Clinical Features of Hypertrophic Cardiomyopathy*

Angina pectoris (relieved by recumbency that decreases left ventricular outflow obstruction)

Left ventricular hypertrophy (vulnerable to myocardial ischemia)

Accelerated coronary atherosclerosis

Syncope

Tachydysrhythmias

Systemic embolism

Congestive heart failure

Cardiac murmur (left ventricular outflow obstruction or mitral regurgitation)

Sudden death

E. **Management of anesthesia** is directed toward minimizing left ventricular outflow obstruction (Table 7-3). Overall, the risk of general anesthesia appears to be acceptable in patients with hypertrophic cardiomyopathy.

1. **Preoperative medication** should ideally decrease anxiety and associated activation of the sympathetic nervous system.

   a. Prophylactic antibiotics may be included in view of the risk of infective endocarditis.

   b. Systemic anticoagulation may be initiated in view of the risk of systemic embolism (this consideration may influence the selection of regional anesthesia).

   c. Expansion of intravascular fluid volume during the preoperative period is important in maintaining intraoperative stroke volume and in minimizing the adverse effects of positive-pressure ventilation of the lungs.

2. **Induction of anesthesia** is designed to avoid sudden drug-induced decreases in systemic vascular resistance. Modest degrees of direct myocardial depression are acceptable (ketamine is an unlikely selection). It is important to minimize activation of the sympathetic nervous system in response to direct laryngoscopy (see Table 5-7).

3. **Maintenance of anesthesia** is designed to produce mild depression of myocardial contractility and, at the same time, preserve intravascular fluid volume and systemic vascular resistance.
   a. Theoretically, halothane, which decreases myocardial contractility more than other volatile anesthetics, would be the preferred selection.
   b. Opioids alone are not likely choices for maintenance of anesthesia, as these drugs do not produce myocardial depression (but may in combination with nitrous oxide).
   c. Peripheral vasodilation, as produced by high levels of sensory anesthesia (spinal or epidural anesthesia), could contribute to increases in left ventricular outflow obstruction.
   d. Nondepolarizing muscle relaxants that have minimal to no effects on the circulation are useful choices.
   e. When intraoperative hypotension occurs, treatment with phenylephrine is recommended (drugs with beta activity may increase myocardial contractility and left ventricular outflow obstruction).
   f. Maintenance of normal sinus rhythm is important, since ventricular filling is dependent on left atrial contraction.

CHAPTER 8

Cor Pulmonale

Cor pulmonale is right ventricular enlargement that develops secondary to pulmonary hypertension (see Stoelting RK, Dierdorf SF. Cor pulmonale. In: Anesthesia and Co-Existing Disease. 3rd Ed. New York. Churchill Livingstone, 1993). Chronic obstructive pulmonary disease (COPD) with associated loss of pulmonary capillaries and arterial hypoxemia leading to pulmonary vascular vasoconstriction is the most likely cause of cor pulmonale. An estimated 10% to 30% of patients (most often males) admitted to the hospital with congestive heart failure (CHF) exhibit cor pulmonale.

I. SIGNS AND SYMPTOMS (Table 8-1)

   A. Clinical manifestations of cor pulmonale are often nonspecific and tend to be obscured by co-existing COPD.
   B. When pulmonary hypertension develops gradually, as with COPD, and the right ventricle has time to compensate, CHF rarely occurs until mean pulmonary artery pressure is >50 mmHg.
      1. In patients with COPD, acute right ventricular failure may develop during pulmonary infections.
      2. This CHF may reverse spontaneously with successful treatment of the pulmonary infection, presumably reflecting a concomitant decrease in pulmonary vascular resistance.

II. TREATMENT (Table 8-2)

   A. The goal is to decrease the workload of the right ventricle by decreasing pulmonary vascular resistance.
   B. This goal is best achieved by returning arterial blood gases (PaO_2 >60 mmHg, SaO_2 >90%) and pH to normal.
   C. Long-term anticoagulation is often recommended as prophylaxis against thrombus formation that may result in pulmonary emboli. A small pulmonary embolism that would have little effect on a normal patient could have catastrophic consequences in a patient with pulmonary hypertension.
   D. Unfortunately, vasodilating drugs often affect the systemic circulation more than the pulmonary circulation.

Table 8-1. *Signs and Symptoms of Cor Pulmonale*

Dyspnea

Effort-related syncope

Mean pulmonary artery pressure >20 mmHg
(>35 mmHg is severe pulmonary artery hypertension)

Accentuation of the pulmonic component of the
second heart sound

Right atrial pressure tracing exhibits prominent A wave

Evidence of overt right ventricular failure (see
Table 6-3)

Table 8-2. *Treatment of Cor Pulmonale*

Supplemental oxygen

Diuretics

Digitalis

Vasodilators

Anticoagulants

Antibiotics

Heart-lung transplantation

III. MANAGEMENT OF ANESTHESIA

A. It is recommended that elective operations in patients
with cor pulmonale be postponed until reversible components of co-existing COPD are treated (Table 8-3).

B. Preoperative determination of arterial blood gases and pH
provide guidelines for management of the patient during
the intraoperative and postoperative period.

C. Induction of anesthesia should avoid abrupt decreases in
systemic vascular resistance in the presence of a fixed
increase in pulmonary vascular resistance.

D. Maintenance of anesthesia is usually achieved with inhala-
tional anesthetics.

1. Enflurane and isoflurane are probably as effective as
halothane as bronchodilators.

2. Nitrous oxide may produce pulmonary artery vasoconstriction.

> **Table 8-3.** *Preoperative Preparation of the Patient With Cor Pulmonale*
>
> Elimination and control of pulmonary infection
> Reversal of bronchospasm
> Improvement of secretion clearance
> Expansion of collapsed or poorly ventilated alveoli
> Hydration
> Correction of electrolyte imbalance

3. Positive-pressure ventilation of the lungs may further increase pulmonary vascular resistance, but this adverse effect is more than offset by improved ventilation-to-perfusion relationships and arterial oxygenation.

4. Hyperventilation-induced metabolic alkalosis resulting in hypokalemia is to be avoided in patients being treated with digitalis.

5. Regional anesthetic techniques that produce a high sensory level are discouraged as a decrease in systemic vascular resistance in the presence of fixed pulmonary hypertension could produce undesirable degrees of systemic hypotension.

E. **Monitoring** of the patient with cor pulmonale is influenced by the invasiveness of the operation.

1. A right atrial catheter gives useful information regarding right ventricular function and the safety of the intravenous infusion of fluids.

2. An abrupt increase in right atrial pressure that signals right ventricular dysfunction may reflect unrecognized arterial hypoxemia, hypoventilation, or the impact of nitrous oxide.

3. When left ventricular dysfunction accompanies cor pulmonale, it may be helpful to place a pulmonary artery catheter rather than a central venous catheter.

IV. PRIMARY PULMONARY HYPERTENSION

A. This is a diagnosis of exclusion when there is no recognizable cause of pulmonary hypertension.

1. There is often evidence of vasospastic disease (Raynaud's

       phenomenon, Prinzmetal's angina, migraine headache).
   2. Primary pulmonary hypertension may present for the first time during pregnancy.
B. Treatment and management of anesthesia are as described for cor pulmonale.

CHAPTER 9

Pericardial Diseases

Pericardial diseases result from diverse causes that evoke responses described as acute pericarditis, pericardial effusion, or chronic constrictive pericarditis (see Stoelting RK, Dierdorf SF. Pericardial diseases. In: Anesthesia and Co-Existing Disease. 3rd Ed. New York. Churchill Livingstone, 1993).

I. ACUTE PERICARDITIS

   A. This is an inflammatory process of the pericardium that may be due to a variety of causes but most often reflects a viral infection (Table 9-1).
   B. **Diagnosis** is suggested by the sudden onset of severe chest pain exaggerated by inspiration, plus diffuse ST segment elevation on the electrocardiogram (presumably reflecting extension of the inflammatory reaction to the surface of the heart).
   C. Treatment is symptomatic, including analgesics and corticosteroids.
   D. Acute pericarditis in the absence of an associated pericardial effusion does not alter cardiac function.

II. PERICARDIAL EFFUSION

   A. Inflammatory reaction characteristic of acute pericarditis may be associated with the accumulation of fluid in the pericardial space.
   B. If the effusion develops gradually, the pericardium can stretch to accommodate a large volume of fluid without a significant increase in pressure, whereas even a small volume of fluid (100 to 200 ml) that accumulates rapidly may cause acute cardiac tamponade.
   C. Echocardiography is the most useful method for clinical detection of a pericardial effusion.

III. CHRONIC CONSTRICTIVE PERICARDITIS

   A. **Diagnosis** of constrictive pericarditis depends on recognition of increased venous pressure in a patient who does not have other obvious evidence of heart disease.
      1. Elevation and eventual equalization (about 20 mmHg) of right atrial pressure, pulmonary artery end-diastolic

Table 9-1. *Causes of Acute Pericarditis With or Without Pericardial Effusion*

Infectious
  Viral
  Bacterial
  Fungal
  Tuberculosis (often associated with acquired immunodeficiency syndrome)

Postmyocardial infarction (Dressler syndrome)

Post-traumatic (cardiac surgery, pacemaker, or pressure-monitoring catheters)

Metastatic disease

Drug-induced (minoxidil, procainamide)

Mediastinal radiation

Systemic disease
  Rheumatoid arthritis
  Systemic lupus erythematosus
  Scleroderma

pressure, and pulmonary artery occlusion pressure may occur in the presence of both chronic constrictive pericarditis and cardiac tamponade.

2. Atrial dysrhythmias are common, presumably reflecting involvement of the sinoatrial node by the disease process.
3. Myocardial function is usually normal.
4. Computed tomography reveals pericardial thickening.

B. Treatment is surgical removal of the constricting adherent pericardium, with the aid of cardiopulmonary bypass if necessary. Hemodynamic improvement (decrease in right atrial pressure) does not occur immediately, in contrast to the prompt improvement that follows treatment of cardiac tamponade.

C. Management of Anesthesia

1. Combinations of benzodiazepines, opioids, and nitrous oxide with or without low doses of volatile anesthetics are acceptable for maintenance of anesthesia (the goal is to avoid decreases in myocardial contractility, blood pressure, heart rate, and venous return).

2. Preoperative optimization of intravascular fluid volume is important.
3. Invasive monitoring of arterial and venous pressure is useful, as removal of adherent pericardium may be associated with decreases in blood pressure and cardiac output.
4. Cardiac dysrhythmias are common during surgical removal of adherent pericardium.

IV. CARDIAC TAMPONADE

A. Cardiac tamponade may be a cause of low cardiac output during the early postoperative period after cardiac surgery. It may necessitate urgent return to the operating room.

B. **Echocardiography** is the most useful method for detecting the presence of pericardial fluid (cardiac silhouette on a chest radiograph does not change until about 250 ml of fluid is present in the pericardial space).

C. **Signs and Symptoms** (Table 9-2)
1. A high index of suspicion is necessary for the prompt diagnosis of cardiac tamponade. Many of the initial manifestations mimic pulmonary embolism.
2. Accumulation of blood and blood clots over the right ventricle, as often occurs after cardiac surgery, may result in selective elevation of right atrial pressure.

Table 9-2. *Signs and Symptoms of Cardiac Tamponade*

Increased central venous pressure

Activation of the sympathetic nervous system (tachycardia, vasoconstriction)

Equalization of atrial filling pressures and pulmonary artery end-diastolic pressure at about 20 mmHg

Decreased voltage and electrical alternans on the electrocardiogram

Paradoxical pulse (systolic blood pressure decrease >10 mmHg during inspiration)

Hypotension

Table 9-3. *Treatment of Cardiac Tamponade*

Measures to Maintain Stroke Volume
  Expansion of intravascular fluid volume (may be necessary to increase right atrial pressure to >25 mmHg)
  Administration of catecholamines (isoproterenol a consideration)
  Correction of metabolic acidosis (sodium bicarbonate 0.5–1 mEq•L^{-1} IV)
  Reverse bradycardia due to vagal reflexes as intrapericardial pressure increases (atropine)
Percutaneous Subxiphoid Pericardiocentesis
Pericardiotomy

    3. Compensatory mechanisms may ultimately fail and **profound hypotension** is likely.

D. Treatment (Table 9-3)

E. Management of Anesthesia

    1. When it is not possible to relieve intrapericardial pressure causing cardiac tamponade before the induction of anesthesia, the goal must be to maintain cardiac output (avoid anesthetic-induced decreases in myocardial contractility, systemic vascular resistance, and heart rate).

      a. Ketamine is useful for induction and maintenance of anesthesia.

      b. Pancuronium is often selected for skeletal muscle relaxation.

    2. It may be prudent to avoid vigorous positive-pressure ventilation of the lungs, as increased intrathoracic pressure can further reduce venous return.

    3. Continuous monitoring of central venous pressure and systemic blood pressure should be initiated before the induction of anesthesia.

    4. Maintenance of elevated central venous pressure with generous administration of intravenous fluids is indicated to maintain venous return.

    5. The ability to perform an emergency pericardiocentesis must be ensured, should circulatory collapse occur after induction of anesthesia.

CHAPTER 10

Aneurysms of the Thoracic and Abdominal Aorta

Diseases of the aorta are most often aneurysmal, whereas occlusive disease is most likely to affect the peripheral arteries (see Stoelting RK, Dierdorf SF. Aneurysms of the thoracic and abdominal aorta. In: Anesthesia and Co-Existing Disease. 3rd Ed. New York. Churchill Livingstone, 1993). The initiating event in aortic dissection is a tear in the intima through which blood surges into a false lumen separating the intima from the adventia for various distances.

I. ANEURYSMS OF THE THORACIC AORTA

A. **Classification.** Aortic dissections can be classified as those that involve the ascending aorta (type A) and those that are limited to the descending aorta (distal to the left subclavian artery) (type B) (Fig. 10-1).

B. **Etiology** (Table 10-1)

C. **Signs and Symptoms** (Table 10-2)

D. **Diagnosis.** Aortic angiography is the most definitive method for confirming the diagnosis of aortic dissection.

E. **Treatment** of aortic dissection reflects an empirical evolution.

1. **Early Short-Term Treatment.** Clinical suspicion of aortic dissection mandates institution of medical therapy, often before diagnostic procedures are initiated (Table 10-3).

2. **Subsequent Definitive Treatment** (Table 10-3)

F. **Management of Anesthesia**

1. Cross-clamping of the thoracic aorta at the suprarenal or supraceliac level is necessary for surgical therapy for a thoracic aneurysm.

a. This cross-clamping is associated with marked increases in systemic vascular resistance and blood pressure, whereas cardiac output declines. Echocardiography often demonstrates abnormal wall motion of the left ventricle, suggesting myocardial ischemia.

b. **Spinal cord ischemia and paraplegia** that accompany aortic cross-clamping presumably reflect inter-

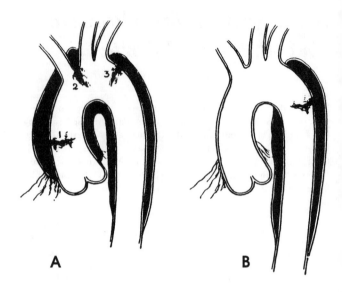

Fig. 10-1. *Aortic dissections may be classified as* **(A)** *those involving the ascending aorta (type A) and* **(B)** *those limited to the descending aorta (type B). The intimal tear in a type A dissection is usually at position 1, whereas the intimal tear for a type B dissection is usually within 2 to 5 cm of the left subclavian artery. (From Daily PO, Trueblook W, Stinson EB, Wuerflein RD, Shumway NE. Management of aortic dissections. Ann Thorac Surg 1970;10:237–47, with permission.)*

Table 10-1. *Etiology of Thoracic Aortic Dissection*

Hypertension (present in 70–90% of afflicted patients)

Congenital disorders of connective tissue
    Marfan syndrome
    Ehlers-Danlos syndrome

Deceleration injuries to the chest

Blunt trauma

Pregnancy

Iatrogenic (site of aortic cannulation or where aorta has been cross-clamped)

Table 10-2. *Signs and Symptoms of Aneurysms of the Thoracic Aorta*

Excruciating chest pain

Diminution or absence of peripheral pulses
Stroke
Paraplegia
Ischemia of extremities

Vasoconstricted and hypertensive

Acute aortic regurgitation

Myocardial infarction

Cardiac tamponade

Table 10-3. *Treatment of Aneurysms of the Thoracic Aorta*

Early Short-Term Treatment
Decrease blood pressure (lower systolic blood pressure to about 100 mmHg using nitroprusside)
Diminish velocity of ventricular contraction (beta antagonist)
Relieve pain

Subsequent Definitive Treatment
Acute proximal aortic dissection (surgical resection with or without aortic valve replacement)
Acute distal thoracic dissection (medical versus surgical therapy)

ruption of the blood supply to the anterior spinal cord. There is no evidence that intraoperative monitoring of somatosensory evoked potentials permits recognition of spinal cord ischemia and avoidance of postoperative neurologic damage.

2. Proper monitoring is more important than the actual drugs selected for anesthesia.

a. Blood pressure should be monitored above (right radial artery or left radial artery if the aneurysm involves the innominate artery) and below (femoral artery) the aneurysm. This approach permits assessment of cerebral perfusion pressure as well as the perfusion pressure to the kidneys during aortic cross-clamping. Attempts are made to maintain the mean arterial pressure close to 100 mmHg in the upper part of the body and >50 mmHg distal to the aneurysm. Use of an external heparinized shunt to bypass the occluded thoracic aorta is a consideration.

    b. Somatosensory evoked potentials or the electroencephalogram are methods with which to evaluate central nervous system viability during aortic cross-clamping.

    c. A pulmonary artery catheter is placed to permit monitoring of cardiac function and adequacy of fluid and blood replacement.

    d. Transesophageal echocardiography may be useful for monitoring left ventricular function during aortic cross-clamping

    e. Diuresis is established preoperatively and maintained intraoperatively with mannitol and/or furosemide.

3. Induction of anesthesia and intubation of the trachea must minimize undesirable increases in blood pressure that could exacerbate the aortic dissection (see Table 5-7). An endobronchial tube permitting collapse of the left lung during resection of the aneurysm is a consideration.

4. General anesthesia, including a volatile anesthetic and opioid, is a frequent selection for maintenance of anesthesia, taking advantage of cerebral metabolic suppression produced by this approach.

G. Postoperative Management

    1. The patient recovering from a thoracic aneurysm resection is at risk of the development of cardiac, ventilatory, and renal failure during the immediate postoperative period.

    2. Cerebrovascular accidents may be produced by air or thrombotic emboli during surgical resection of the diseased aorta.

    3. Spinal cord injury during the postoperative period may manifest as paresis or flaccid paralysis.

    4. Hypertension is not uncommon. It may jeopardize the vascular integrity of the surgical repair and predispose to myocardial ischemia (relieve pain and institute antihypertensive therapy with vasodilators and/or beta antagonists).

II. CARDIAC CONTUSION

A. Deceleration injuries involving the anterior chest wall (right ventricle because of its immediate substernal location) are the most frequent cause of myocardial contusion.

1. Cardiac dysrhythmias and congestive heart failure are the two principal consequences of myocardial contusion. Continuous monitoring of the electrocardiogram is necessary to detect life-threatening ventricular cardiac dysrhythmias, ST and T wave abnormalities, and bundle branch block.

2. **Treatment** of myocardial contusion is symptomatic.

III. ANEURYSMS OF THE ABDOMINAL AORTA

A. An abdominal aneurysm can usually be detected as a pulsating abdominal mass. Confirmation is provided by ultrasound examination.

B. **Treatment** is elective resection and replacement with a prosthetic graft (mortality <5%, with death usually related to myocardial infarction) of any aneurysm >5 cm in diam**eter.**

1. Infrarenal aortic cross-clamping and unclamping is an integral component of abdominal aortic surgery.

a. Deepening anesthesia or administration of a vasodilator during infrarenal aortic occlusion may be necessary in some patients. Nevertheless, myocardial performance and circulatory variables usually remain within an acceptable range after the aorta is occluded at an infrarenal level, even in patients with co-existing cardiac dysfunction.

b. Despite the usually negligible cardiovascular effects of infrarenal aortic cross-clamping, hypotension (transient decreases in systolic blood pressure of about 40 mmHg) may occur when the cross-clamp is removed. Blood pressure changes are minimized by gradual removal of the clamp and by prior volume loading. The role of the washout of acid metabolites from the ischemic extremities when the clamp is released has been discredited as a cause of declamping hypotension.

c. Acute renal failure may follow infrarenal aortic cross-clamping, although maintenance of intravascular fluid volume usually is protective.

C. Management of Anesthesia

1. Preoperative evaluation must consider the high incidence of associated ischemic heart disease, hypertension, and renal dysfunction in these (usually elderly) patients.

2. Monitors during the perioperative period include an intra-arterial catheter and pulmonary artery catheter (it is not possible to predict whether central venous pressure will parallel left heart filling pressure). Transesophageal echocardiography may be a useful monitor of the cardiac response to aortic cross-clamping and unclamping.

3. Combination of a volatile drug and opioid (produces low blood pressure and decreases myocardial oxygen demand) is often selected for maintenance of anesthesia. A vasodilator or inotrope may be required, depending on the intraoperative blood pressure and cardiac output response.

   a. Continuous epidural anesthesia may be combined with a general anesthetic, providing the advantages of attenuation of increased systemic vascular resistance with aortic cross-clamping and alleviation of postoperative pain.

   b. Anticoagulation during abdominal aortic surgery introduces the controversy regarding the placement of an epidural catheter and the remote risk of epidural hematoma formation (see Chapter 25, section IV B).

4. A balanced salt solution, with or without a colloid solution, should be infused during the aortic cross-clamp period to maintain the pulmonary artery occlusion pressure 3 to 5 mmHg above the preclamp value, so as to minimize declamping hypotension and decreased cardiac output.

   a. If urine output is <50 ml·h^{-1} despite adequate fluid and blood replacement, diuretic therapy with mannitol or furosemide may be considered. Low-dose dopamine may also be administered in an attempt to improve renal function.

   b. There is no evidence that drug-induced diuresis is beneficial.

5. The greatest blood loss during elective abdominal aortic aneurysm resection usually occurs when the

aneurysm is opened and lumbar arteries are back-bleeding. Intraoperative blood salvage and reinfusion and acceptance of modest degrees of hemodilution have decreased the need for homologous blood transfusion.

D. Postoperative Management

1. Patients recovering from abdominal aneurysm resection are at risk of the development of cardiac (myocardial ischemia or infarction), ventilatory, and renal failure during the immediate postoperative period.

2. Assessment of graft patency and lower extremity blood flow is important.

3. Hypertension may reflect overzealous intraoperative hydration and/or postoperative hypothermia with compensatory vasoconstriction. Treatment with vasodilators may be necessary.

4. Provision of adequate analgesia as with neuraxial opioids should be given priority.

CHAPTER 11

Peripheral Vascular Disease

Peripheral vascular disease may manifest as systemic vasculitis or arterial occlusive disease (Table 11-1) (see Stoelting RK, Dierdorf SF. Peripheral vascular disease. In: Anesthesia and Co-Existing Disease. 3rd Ed. New York. Churchill Livingstone, 1993). Clinical syndromes involving inflammation of blood levels present in non-specific ways (Table 11-2). Acute peripheral arterial occlusion is most often due to an embolus, whereas chronic occlusion generally reflects atherosclerosis.

I. TAKAYASU'S ARTERITIS

A. Chronic inflammation of the aorta and its major branches (pulseless disease) is reflected by multiple organ dysfunction, most often in Asian females (Table 11-3).

B. Management of Anesthesia

1. Supplemental corticosteroids may be required in patients being treated with these drugs.

2. Regional anesthesia may be controversial in patients being treated with anticoagulants.

3. Blood pressure may be difficult to measure noninvasively in the upper extremities. Despite a theoretical concern, placement of a catheter in the radial artery may be useful.

4. It is important to recognize that hyperextension of the head, as during direct laryngoscopy for intubation of the trachea, may compromise blood flow through carotid arteries that are shortened because of the vascular inflammatory process. During preoperative evaluation, it is useful to establish the effect of changes in head position on cerebral function.

5. Regardless of the drugs selected to produce anesthesia, the priority must be to maintain adequate perfusion pressure during the intraoperative period.

II. THROMBOANGIITIS OBLITERANS

A. Inflammatory and occlusive disease involves arteries and veins of the extremities (intermittent claudication), most often in Jewish males aged 20 to 40 years.

B. Treatment consists of cessation of smoking, avoidance of

Table 11-1. *Peripheral Vascular Disease*

Systemic Vasculitis
  Takayasu's arteritis (pulseless disease)
  Thromboangiitis obliterans (Buerger's disease)
  Wegener's granulomatosis
  Temporal arteritis
  Polyarteritis nodosa
  Schönlein-Henoch purpura
  Raynaud's phenomenon
  Moyamoya disease
  Kawasaki disease

Acute Peripheral Arterial Occlusive Disease (Embolism)

Chronic Peripheral Arterial Occlusive Disease
  (Atherosclerosis)
  Distal abdominal aorta or iliac arteries
  Femoral arteries
  Subclavian steal syndrome
  Coronary-subclavian steal syndrome

Table 11-2. *Signs and Symptoms of Systemic Vasculitis*

Fever
Fatigue
Weight loss
Neuropathy
Increased erythrocyte sedimentation rate
Anemia
Hypoalbuminemia

---

exposure to cold ambient temperatures, administration of vasodilating drugs, and sympathectomy.

C. **Management of Anesthesia**
  1. Positioning during surgery must consider the risk of damage to ischemic extremities.
  2. Raising the ambient temperature of the operating room may be useful.
  3. Noninvasive monitoring of blood pressure is preferred.

Table 11-3. *Signs and Symptoms of Takayasu's Arteritis*

Central Nervous System
  Vertigo
  Visual disturbances
  Syncope
  Seizures
  Cerebral ischemia or infarction

Cardiovascular System
  Multiple occlusions of peripheral arteries
  Ischemic heart disease
  Cardiac valve dysfunction
  Cardiac conduction defects

Lungs
  Pulmonary hypertension
  Ventilation-to-perfusion mismatch

Kidneys
  Renal artery stenosis

Musculoskeletal System
  Ankylosing spondylitis
  Rheumatoid arthritis

III. WEGENER'S GRANULOMATOSIS

  A. This disease is characterized by pathophysiologic changes caused by the formation of necrotizing granulomas in inflamed vessels present in multiple organ systems (Table 11-4).

  B. **Treatment** with cyclophosphamide usually produces dramatic remissions.

  C. **Management of Anesthesia**

  1. Potential adverse effects of cyclophosphamide (depression of the immune system, anemia, decreased plasma cholinesterase activity) are considerations in the preoperative evaluation. Likewise, widespread organ involvement may influence the choice of anesthetic drugs (myocardial ischemia, renal failure) or technique (peripheral neuropathy) (Table 11-4).

  2. Avoidance of trauma during direct laryngoscopy (bleeding from granulomas and dislodgement of fri-

Table 11-4. *Signs and Symptoms of Wegener's Granulomatosis*

Central Nervous System
  Cerebral arterial aneurysms
  Peripheral neuropathy

Respiratory Tract and Lungs
  Sinusitis
  Laryngeal stenosis
  Epiglottic destruction
  Ventilation-to-perfusion mismatch
  Pneumonia
  Hemoptysis
  Bronchial destruction

Cardiovascular System
  Cardiac valve destruction
  Disturbances of cardiac impulse conduction
  Myocardial ischemia
  Infarction of the tips of digits

Kidneys
  Hematuria
  Azotemia
  Renal failure

able tissues) and the use of a smaller than expected endotracheal tube are important considerations.

3. Arteritis that is likely to involve peripheral vessels may limit the placement of an indwelling arterial catheter to monitor blood pressure.

IV. TEMPORAL ARTERITIS

A. Any patient over 50 years of age complaining of a unilateral headache is suspect for this diagnosis.

B. Superficial branches of the temporal arteries are often tender and enlarged. Arteritis of branches of the ophthalmic artery may lead to ischemic optic neuritis and sudden blindness, unless treated promptly with corticosteroids.

V. POLYARTERITIS NODOSA

A. Small and medium-size arteries are involved with inflammatory changes, resulting in glomerulitis, myocardial ischemia, peripheral neuropathies, and seizures, most often in females 20 to 60 years of age and commonly in association with allergic reactions to drugs.

B. Renal failure with associated hypertension is the most common cause of death.

C. **Management of anesthesia** should take into consideration the likelihood of renal and cardiac disease, as well as adverse effects of drugs (cyclophosphamide, corticosteroids) used to treat this disease.

VI. RAYNAUD'S PHENOMENON

A. This disease is characterized by cold-induced arterial spasm in the extremities, manifesting most often in adult females and invariably in the presence of underlying disease (scleroderma, systemic lupus erythematosus).

B. Arterial spasm and pain may be relieved on occasion by intravenous administration of reserpine or guanethidine into a tourniquet-isolated extremity. In severe cases, interruption of the sympathetic nervous system supply to the hand may be considered (stellate ganglion block).

C. **Management of Anesthesia**

   1. Maintaining body temperature and increasing the ambient temperature of the operating room are important considerations.

   2. Blood pressure is most often monitored by a noninvasive technique, in view of the theoretical risk of placing a catheter in a peripheral artery supplying a potentially ischemic extremity.

   3. Regional anesthesia is acceptable, but it is prudent not to include epinephrine in the local anesthetic solution.

VII. MOYAMOYA DISEASE

A. This disease is characterized by narrowing or occlusion of both internal carotid arteries, manifesting most often as transient ischemic attacks (children) or as intracerebral hemorrhage from an intracranial aneurysm (adults).

B. **Management of anesthesia** must preserve a balance between cerebral blood flow and cerebral oxygen requirements, which may be adversely altered by spinal anesthesia in these patients.

1. Isoflurane has been recommended because of its mild cerebral vasodilating effects and ability to greatly decrease cerebral metabolic rate.
2. The presence of neurologic changes may limit the use of succinylcholine.

VIII. KAWASAKI DISEASE

A. This disease manifests as fever, conjunctivitis, cervical lymphadenopathy, and vasculitis (involving walls of coronary arteries, often leading to aneurysmal dilation) in children.
B. Complications include myocardial infarction and cerebral hemorrhage.

IX. ACUTE PERIPHERAL ARTERIAL OCCLUSIVE DISEASE

A. Manifestations occur most commonly in the extremities, reflecting lodgment of an embolus at an arterial bifurcation. The result is sudden pain and sharply demarcated skin color changes below the level of the arterial occlusion.
B. Surgical embolectomy and adjunctive heparin therapy are recommended when an acute embolism lodges in a large peripheral artery and causes persistent ischemia.

X. CHRONIC PERIPHERAL ARTERIAL OCCLUSIVE DISEASE

A. This disease is almost always due to peripheral atherosclerosis (diffuse, as in the elderly patient with diabetes mellitus, versus segmental). It often occurs in association with coronary or cerebral atherosclerosis.
  1. Occlusion of the distal abdominal aorta or iliac arteries tends to occur in males <60 years of age and manifests as claudication in the hips and buttocks.
  2. Occlusion of the common femoral or superficial femoral arteries is the most common form of segmental peripheral atherosclerosis, especially in elderly patients. It produces a syndrome of claudication in or below the calf.
B. **Treatment** includes revascularization procedures, such as femorofemoral bypass and femoropopliteal bypass.

Lumbar sympathectomy may contribute to graft patency during the early postoperative period. Antiplatelet therapy is often begun preoperatively.

C. Management of Anesthesia

1. The principal risk of anesthesia for revascularization procedures is associated ischemic heart disease.

2. The popularity of general anesthesia is in part due to the controversy surrounding the performance of regional anesthesia, especially placement of a lumbar epidural catheter, in the presence of drug-induced anticoagulation (see Chapter 25, section IV B).

   a. Nevertheless, placement of an epidural catheter before instituting heparin anticoagulation has not been associated with untoward neurologic events.

   b. Epidural analgesia may beneficially influence outcome (attenuates stress-induced hypercoagulability) in high-risk patients, following major peripheral vascular surgery.

3. Infrarenal aortic cross-clamping and unclamping in the presence of peripheral vascular disease is associated with minimal hemodynamic derangements, presumably reflecting the presence of collateral circulation. For this reason, it may be acceptable to use a central venous pressure catheter in lieu of a pulmonary artery catheter.

4. Thromboembolic complications, especially in the kidneys, most likely reflect dislodgment of atheroembolic debris from the diseased aorta. Gentle surgical handling is more protective than heparin.

5. Spinal cord damage is unlikely, and special monitoring is not necessary.

D. Subclavian Steal Syndrome

1. Occlusion of the subclavian or innominate artery proximal to the origin of the vertebral artery by an atherosclerotic lesion may result in reversal of flow (steal) from the brain (syncope).

2. There is often an absent or diminished pulse in the ipsilateral arm. The systolic blood pressure is likely to be at least 20 mmHg lower in the ipsilateral arm.

E. Coronary-Subclavian Steal Syndrome

1. This syndrome occurs when incomplete stenosis of the left subclavian artery leads to reversal of blood flow (steal) through a patent internal mammary artery

graft. It is manifested as angina pectoris and decreased systolic blood pressure of at least 20 mmHg in the ipsilateral arm.

2. Bilateral upper extremity brachial artery blood pressure measurement may be useful in the preoperative evaluation of patients with an internal mammary to coronary artery bypass graft.

CHAPTER 12

Deep Vein Thrombosis and Pulmonary Embolism

Deep vein thrombosis (formation of clot in a blood vessel) and associated pulmonary embolism (fragment of a thrombus that breaks off and travels in the blood) are among the leading causes of postoperative morbidity and mortality (see Stoelting RK, Dierdorf SF. Deep vein thrombosis and pulmonary embolism. In: Anesthesia and Co-Existing Disease. 3rd Ed. New York. Churchill Livingstone, 1993). Factors that predispose to thromboembolism are multiple but often include events likely to be associated with anesthesia and surgery (Table 12-1).

I. DEEP VEIN THROMBOSIS

A. Venous thrombi that form below the knees or in the arms rarely give rise to significant pulmonary emboli, whereas thrombi that extend into the ileofemoral venous system can produce life-threatening pulmonary embolism.

B. Diagnosis and Treatment

1. **Superficial thrombophlebitis,** as may follow an intravenous infusion, is rarely associated with pulmonary embolism (intense inflammation leads to rapid and total occlusion of the vein). Treatment of superficial vein thrombosis is conservative (elevation, heat, antibiotics if infection suspected).

2. Deep Vein Thrombosis

a. **Diagnosis** on the basis of clinical signs (throbbing pain, edema) is unreliable and venography may demonstrate negative results despite subsequent occurrence of pulmonary embolism. **Ultrasound** is a highly sensitive noninvasive method for detecting proximal deep vein thrombi (ileofemoral).

b. **Heparin** (5000 units IV), followed by a continuous intravenous infusion adjusted to maintain the activated partial thromboplastin time 1.5 to 2 times normal for 10 days, is the accepted treatment of proximal deep vein thrombosis.

c. **Complications.** Intracranial hemorrhage, thrombocytopenia, and increased serum aminotransferase concentrations are possible side effects of heparin

Table 12-1. *Predisposing Factors to Thromboembolism*

Venous Stasis
Trauma (including surgery)
Lack of ambulation
Pregnancy
Low cardiac output (congestive heart failure, myocardial infarction)

Abnormality of Venous Wall
Varicose veins
Drug-induced irritation

Hypercoagulable State
Estrogen therapy (oral contraceptives)
Cancer (Trousseau syndrome)
Deficiencies of endogenous anticoagulants (antithrombin III, protein C, protein S)
Stress response associated with surgery

History of Previous Thromboembolism

Morbid Obesity

Advanced Age

therapy. Nevertheless, the only absolute contraindication to the use of heparin is the presence of a known coagulation disorder or active hemorrhage.

C. **Prophylaxis**
   1. Venous stasis is minimized by exercise (flexion and extension at the knees) and by the use of elastic stockings applied preoperatively.
   2. **Subcutaneous heparin** (5000 units every 12 hours) initiated preoperatively has been demonstrated to prevent about two-thirds of all deep vein thromboses and about one-half of all pulmonary emboli among patients undergoing urologic, orthopaedic, or general surgical procedures. Institution of preoperative subcutaneous heparin therapy introduces concern regarding the subsequent use of regional anesthesia and the possibility of hematoma formation, especially in the epidural space.
   3. **Regional anesthesia** may decrease the postoperative incidence of deep vein thrombosis and pulmonary embolism, compared with the same surgery performed with general anesthesia.

II. PULMONARY EMBOLISM

A. Clinical manifestations of pulmonary embolism are non-specific. The diagnosis is often difficult to establish on clinical grounds alone (Table 12-2).

1. Arterial blood gases that accompany pulmonary embolism are characterized by decreased PaO_2 and $PaCO_2$.

2. Changes on the electrocardiogram are unlikely in the absence of a pulmonary embolism sufficient to cause acute cor pulmonale.

3. Manifestations of pulmonary embolism during anesthesia are nonspecific (unexplained arterial hypoxemia, hypotension, tachycardia, bronchospasm) and often transient.

B. **Diagnosis** of pulmonary embolism may require both non-invasive (ventilation-to-perfusion scans) and invasive (pulmonary arteriography) tests.

C. **Treatment** of pulmonary embolism is intended to support cardiopulmonary function (catecholamines, intubation of the trachea, and mechanical support of ventilation) and to prevent extension or recurrence of the embolus (heparin).

1. Isoproterenol is an attractive but unproven superior

Table 12-2. *Signs and Symptoms of Pulmonary Embolism*

Sign/Symptom	Patients (%)
Acute dyspnea	80–85
Tachypnea (>20 breaths·min^{-1})	75–85
Pleuritic chest pain	65–70
Nonproductive cough	50–60
Accentuation of pulmonic valve second sound	50–60
Rales	50–60
Tachycardia (>100 beats·min^{-1})	45–65
Fever (38°–39°C)	40–50
Hemoptysis	30

choice, as it is more likely than other catecholamines to decrease pulmonary vascular resistance.

2. Since more than 90% of pulmonary emboli originate from thrombi in the legs, surgical treatment may include placement of an umbrella filter in the inferior vena cava.

3. Pulmonary artery embolectomy using cardiopulmonary bypass is reserved for the patient with massive pulmonary embolism who is unresponsive to medical therapy.

4. An analgesic to treat pain associated with pulmonary embolism is important. However, it must be prescribed keeping in mind the underlying instability of the cardiovascular system.

D. **Management of anesthesia** for the surgical treatment of life-threatening pulmonary embolism is designed to support vital organ function and minimize anesthetic-induced myocardial depression.

1. Monitoring of arterial and cardiac filling pressures is used to optimize fluid replacement and titrate inotropic support of cardiac function.

2. Drugs that may increase pulmonary vascular resistance (ketamine, nitrous oxide) are generally avoided. However, other beneficial effects of ketamine may make this drug a useful selection.

3. Pancuronium is an acceptable drug for induction of skeletal muscle paralysis.

4. Removal of emboli fragments from the distal pulmonary arteries may be facilitated by the application of positive-pressure ventilation of the lungs, as when the

---

Table 12-3. *Signs and Symptoms of Fat Embolism*

Arterial hypoxemia (may be the only manifestation)

Adult respiratory distress syndrome

Central nervous system dysfunction (confusion, coma, seizures)

Petechiae (neck, shoulders, and chest)

Coagulopathy

Fever

surgeon applies suction through the arteriotomy placed in the pulmonary trunk.

III. FAT EMBOLISM

A. The syndrome of fat embolism to the lungs typically appears 12 to 48 hours after a long bone fracture, especially of the femur or tibia (Table 12-3).

B. **Treatment** is supportive, with administration of corticosteroids and immobilization of long bone fractures.

CHAPTER 13

Chronic Obstructive Pulmonary Disease

Chronic obstructive pulmonary disease (COPD) affects an estimated 10 million Americans and is most often due to tobacco abuse (see Stoelting RK, Dierdorf SF. Chronic obstructive pulmonary disease. In: Anesthesia and Co-Existing Disease. 3rd Ed. New York. Churchill Livingstone, 1993). These patients are extraordinarily vulnerable to development of acute respiratory failure from insults (acute respiratory infections, surgery) that would not affect normal individuals. Asthma is distinguished from COPD on the basis of a reversible component of airway obstruction (see Chapter 14).

I. CHRONIC BRONCHITIS AND PULMONARY EMPHYSEMA

A. **Epidemiology.** Cigarette smoking is the major predisposing factor in the development of COPD.

1. The dominant feature of the natural history of COPD is progressive airflow obstruction, as reflected by decreases in the forced exhaled volume in 1 second(FEV_1).

2. **Emphysema** may develop in some patients because of an imbalance between protease and antiprotease activities **(alpha-1-antitrypsin deficiency)** in the lungs. Cirrhosis of the liver may also be present in these patients.

B. **Clinical Features and Diagnosis** (Table 13-1)

1. **Chronic productive cough and progressive exercise limitation** (dyspnea that occurs while climbing one flight of stairs or less) are the hallmarks of persistent expiratory airflow obstruction (FEV_1 <80%) characteristic of COPD.

2. Measurement of lung volumes typically indicates increased residual volume and functional residual capacity (FRC) (Fig. 13-1).

3. **Radiographic abnormalities** (hyperlucency and hyperinflation of the lungs, bullae) may be minimal, even in the presence of advanced COPD.

4. **Arterial blood gases** are commonly used to categorize the patient as a "pink puffer" (PaO_2 >60 mmHg, $PaCO_2$ normal) or a "blue bloater" (PaO_2 <60 mmHg, $PaCO_2$ >45 mmHg) (Table 13-1). In the absence of arterial hypoxemia ("pink puffer"), there is little stimulus to

Table 13-1. *Comparative Features of Chronic Obstructive Pulmonary Disease*

	Chronic Bronchitis	**Pulmonary Emphysema**
Mechanism of airway obstruction	Decreased airway lumen due to mucus and inflammation	Loss of elastic recoil
Dyspnea	Moderate	Severe
Forced exhaled volume in 1 second	Decreased	Decreased
PaO_2	Marked decrease ("blue bloater")	Modest decrease ("pink puffer")
$PaCO_2$	Increased	Normal to decreased
Diffusing capacity	Normal	Decreased
Hematocrit	Increased	Normal
Cor pulmonale	Marked	Mild
Prognosis	Poor	Good

pulmonary vasoconstriction (cor pulmonale unlikely), and secondary erythropoiesis does not develop.

C. Treatment consists of cessation of smoking and chronic administration of supplemental oxygen to those patients with a PaO_2 <60 mmHg, a hematocrit >35%, or evidence of cor pulmonale (relief of arterial hypoxemia is more effective than any other drug therapy in decreasing pulmonary vascular resistance).

D. **Preoperative evaluation** of patients with COPD should determine the severity of the disease and elucidate any reversible components such as bronchospasm or infection (Table 13-2). The likelihood of postoperative pulmonary complications is increased in the patient with COPD, associated preoperatively with sputum production and decreased vital capacity and/or FEV_1.

E. **Management of Anesthesia**

1. **Regional anesthesia** is most suited for operations that do not invade the peritoneum (sensory level below T6) or surgical procedures performed on the extremities. Sedation must be titrated as these patients may be extremely sensitive to ventilatory depressant effects of injected drugs.

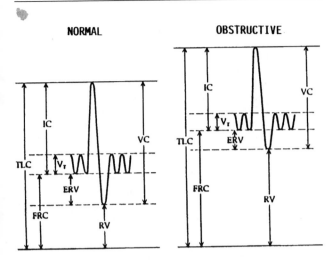

Fig. 13-1. *Lung volumes in chronic obstructive pulmonary disease compared with normal values. In the presence of obstructive lung disease, VC is normal to decreased, RV and FRC are increased, TLC is normal to increased, and RV/TLC ratio is increased. TLC, total lung capacity; FRC, functional residual capacity; RV, residual volume; VC, vital capacity; V_T, tidal volume; IC, inspiratory capacity; ERV, expiratory reserve volume.*

Table 13-2. *Preoperative Evaluation of the Patient With Chronic Obstructive Pulmonary Disease*

Pulmonary function tests (reflect ability to clear secretions; FEV_1/FVC <0.5 suggests increased risk of postoperative respiratory failure)

Arterial blood gases ($PaCO_2$ >50 suggests increased risk of postoperative respiratory failure)

Eradication of acute bacterial infection (purulent sputum suggests acute infection)

Familiarization with respiratory therapy equipment

Cessation of cigarette smoking (carboxyhemoglobin levels decrease in 12–18 hours; improvement in ciliary and small airway function and decreases in sputum production require weeks)

2. **General anesthesia** in a patient with COPD is often provided with a volatile anesthetic (rapid elimination minimizes residual ventilatory depression, drug-induced bronchodilation) using humidification of the inspired gases and mechanical ventilation of the lungs (large tidal volume and slow breathing rate).

   a. Nitrous oxide is often administered with the volatile anesthetic. It should be recognized that this gas could lead to enlargement and rupture of bullae (tension pneumothorax), as well as limiting the inspired concentration of oxygen.

   b. Opioids, although acceptable, may be associated with prolonged depression of ventilation.

   c. A large tidal volume (10 to 15 ml·kg^{-1}) optimizes the matching of ventilation to perfusion, whereas a slow breathing rate (6 to 10 breaths·min^{-1}) provides sufficient time for complete exhalation; this is particularly important if air trapping is to be minimized in patients with COPD. This pattern of mechanical ventilation is often as efficacious as positive end-expiratory pressure with respect to arterial oxygenation, without the detrimental cardiovascular effects produced by sustained positive airway pressure.

   d. Regardless of the method of ventilation of the lungs selected during surgery, objective adjustments in the mode of ventilation or in ventilator settings can be made only on the basis of continuous monitoring of oxygen saturation (pulse oximetry) and end-tidal carbon dioxide concentration (capnography), combined with intermittent measurement of arterial blood gases.

F. **Postoperative care** of the patient with COPD is intended to minimize the incidence and severity of pulmonary complications. It should be recognized that these patients are at increased risk of the development of acute respiratory failure.

   1. Postoperative **pulmonary complications** are most often characterized by atelectasis, followed by pneumonia and decreases in the PaO_2 (Fig. 13-2).

   2. Upper abdominal surgery is associated with the greatest decrease in FRC and PaO_2, and thus the highest incidence of postoperative pulmonary complications.

   3. Choice of drugs or techniques used to produce anes-

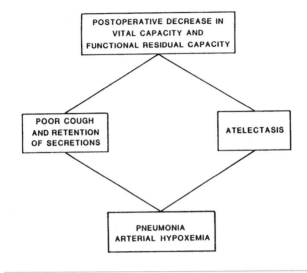

Fig. 13-2. *Pathogenesis of postoperative pulmonary complications.*

thesia does not seem to alter predictably the incidence of postoperative pulmonary complications.

4. **Prophylaxis against pulmonary complications** is based on restoring decreased lung volumes (FRC the most important) and facilitating the production of an effective cough so as to remove secretions from the airways (Table 13-3).

II. BRONCHIECTASIS

A. Localized and irreversible dilation of a bronchus by destructive inflammatory processes is visible on computed tomography.

B. Productive cough of purulent secretions is suggestive of the diagnosis.

C. **Treatment** consists of antibiotics and postural drainage. Bronchial artery embolization may be useful in severe cases of hemoptysis.

D. **Management of anesthesia** may include use of a double-lumen endobronchial tube to prevent spillage of purulent sputum into normal areas of the lungs. Instrumentation of

Table 13-3. *Prophylaxis Against Pulmonary Complications*

Continued intubation of the trachea and mechanical ventilation of the lungs (maintain PaO_2 60–100 mmHg and $PaCO_2$ in range that results in a pH of 7.35–7.45; positive end-expiratory pressure a consideration if cannot maintain PaO_2 >60 mmHg breathing 50% oxygen)

Analgesia (neuraxial opioids permit early tracheal extubation and ambulation)

Chest physiotherapy and postural drainage

Voluntary deep breathing (maintain peak inflation for 3–5 seconds)

Incentive spirometry

Intermittent positive-pressure breathing (efficacy inconclusive; emphasis should be on tidal volume rather than on peak inspiratory pressure)

the nares may not be prudent, in view of the high incidence of chronic sinusitis.

III. CYSTIC FIBROSIS

A. This is an inherited disease characterized by a defect in exocrine gland secretion, leading to production of chemically abnormal sweat and viscous mucus (chloride concentrations >60 mEq·L^{-1}).

1. Impaired clearance of viscous secretions leads to mucous plugging of the airways with resulting obstruction to expiratory airflow, dyspnea, productive cough, and secondary bacterial infection.

2. Extrapulmonary manifestations of cystic fibrosis include pancreatic insufficiency, cirrhosis of the liver, and gastrointestinal obstruction (meconium ileus, vitamin K deficiency).

B. **Management of Anesthesia** (see section I E)

1. Elective surgical procedures should be delayed until optimal pulmonary function can be ensured by control of bronchial infection and facilitation of the removal of secretions from the airways.

2. A volatile anesthetic is helpful in reducing responsive-

ness of the hyperreactive airways characteristic of cystic fibrosis.

3. Frequent suctioning of the trachea is often necessary during the operative period.

IV. KARTAGENER SYNDROME is an inherited trait characterized by situs inversus, chronic sinusitis, and bronchiectasis.

A. Management of Anesthesia

1. In the presence of dextrocardia, it is necessary to reverse placement of the electrocardiographic leads. Inversion of the major vasculature should prompt the recommendation of left internal jugular vein cannulation or right uterine displacement in the parturient.

2. Inversion of the lungs is an indication to use a left double-lumen endobronchial tube with the bronchial portion directed into the right mainstem bronchus.

V. BRONCHIOLITIS OBLITERANS as a cause of chronic airflow obstruction may accompany viral pneumonia and collagen vascular disease (rheumatoid arthritis); it may be a side effect of bone marrow transplantation.

VI. TRACHEAL STENOSIS

A. Prolonged translaryngeal intubation of the trachea or tracheostomy may produce tracheal mucosal scarring and constricting scar formation (symptoms when lumen of the adult trachea is <5 mm).

1. Dyspnea is prominent even at rest.

2. The flow-volume loop is likely to reveal flattened exhaled and inhaled portions (see Fig. 14-2), whereas tomograms of the trachea demonstrate tracheal narrowing.

B. **Treatment** may require surgical resection of the stenotic tracheal segment.

1. Initially, a translaryngeal tracheal tube is placed, followed by insertion of a sterile cuffed tube after exposure of the distal normal trachea.

2. Helium added to the inspired gases may improve gas flow through the area of tracheal narrowing.

3. Maintenance of anesthesia is with a volatile anesthetic to ensure a maximum inspired concentration of oxygen.

CHAPTER 14

Bronchial Asthma

Bronchial asthma is a disease defined by the presence of (1) increased responsiveness of the airways to various stimuli, (2) reversible expiratory airflow obstruction, and (3) chronic inflammatory changes in the submucosa of the airways (see Stoelting RK, Dierdorf SF. Bronchial Asthma. In: Anesthesia and Co-Existing Disease. 3rd Ed. New York. Churchill Livingstone, 1993). There is no pathognomonic feature or definitive diagnostic test, although a greater than 15% increase in expiratory airflow in response to bronchodilator therapy is supportive evidence when asthma is suspected on clinical grounds. It is estimated that 3% to 6% of the United States population is affected by asthma.

I. PATHOGENESIS (Tables 14-1 and 14-2)

II. SIGNS AND SYMPTOMS

A. During periods of normal to near-normal pulmonary function, patients are likely to have no physical findings referable to their asthma.

B. As expiratory airflow obstruction increases, a number of signs and symptoms may manifest and offer clues as to the severity of the asthmatic attack (Table 14-3).

1. The forced exhaled volume in 1 second (FEV_1) and the maximum midexpiratory flow rate are direct reflections of the severity of expiratory airflow obstruction (Fig. 14-1 and Table 14-4).

2. The flow-volume loop demonstrates a characteristic downward scooping of the expiratory limb of the loop (Fig. 14-2).

3. Mild asthma is usually accompanied by a normal PaO_2 and $PaCO_2$ (Table 14-4).

III. CLASSIFICATION (Table 14-5)

IV. TREATMENT

A. Conceptually, treatment of asthma is with drugs classified as bronchodilators (acute exacerbations) and anti-inflammatory drugs (prophylaxis) (Table 14-6).

1. Serial determinations of pulmonary function are useful for monitoring the response to treatment.

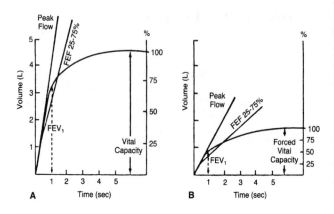

Fig. 14-1. *Spirogram changes of **(A)** a normal subject and **(B)** a patient in bronchospasm. The forced exhaled volume in 1 second (FEV_1) is typically less than 80% of the vital capacity in the presence of obstructive airway disease. Peak flow and maximum midexpiratory flow rate ($FEF_{25-75\%}$) are also decreased in these patients (Fig. B). (From Kingston HGG, Hirshman CA. Perioperative management of the patient with asthma. Anesth Analg 1984;63:844–55, with permission.)*

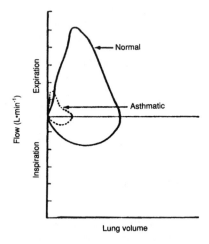

Fig. 14-2. *Flow-volume curve of a normal and of an asthmatic patient. (From Kingston HGG, Hirshman CA. Perioperative management of the patient with asthma. Anesth Analg 1984;63:844–55, with permission.)*

Table 14-1. *Pathogenesis of Asthma*

Release of chemical mediators (histamine, leukotrienes, prostaglandins)

Abnormalities of autonomic nervous system regulation of airway tone (imbalance between excitatory and inhibitory tone)

Chronic airway inflammatory response

Table 14-2. *Precipitating Factors for Acute Asthma*

Inhaled or ingested antigens

Strenuous exercise

Viral upper respiratory tract infections

Inhaled irritants

Reflux of acidic gastric fluid into the lower esophagus

Table 14-3. *Signs and Symptoms of Asthma*

Wheezing (most common finding during an acute asthma attack)

Cough

Dyspnea (parallels severity of expiratory airflow obstruction)

Tachypnea

Table 14-4. *Severity of Expiratory Airflow Obstruction*

	$FEV_1{}^a$ (% Predicted)	$FEF_{25-75\%}{}^a$ (% Predicted)	$PaO_2{}^b$ (mmHg)	$PaCO_2{}^b$ (mmHg)
Mild (asymptomatic)	65–80	60–75	>60	<40
Moderate	50–64	45–59	>60	<45
Marked	35–49	30–44	<60	>50
Severe (status asthmaticus)	<35	<30	<60	>50

[a] See Fig. 14-1 for definitions.
[b] Values are estimates.

Table 14-5. *Classification of Asthma*

Allergen-induced (often associated with allergic rhinitis)

Exercise-induced (decrease in airway temperature may evoke symptoms)

Nocturnal

Aspirin-induced (nasal polyps)

Occupational

Infectious

Table 14-6. *Treatment of Asthma*

Bronchodilator Drugs
 Beta-2 agonists (albuterol by metered dose inhaler)

 Theophylline (5 mg•kg^{-1} IV, followed by 0.5–1 mg•kg^{-1}•h^{-1}; side effects may include cardiac dysrhythmias and seizures)

 Anticholinergics (ipratropium by metered dose inhaler)

Anti-inflammatory Drugs
 Corticosteroids (systemic effects or adrenal gland suppression do not occur with delivery by metered dose inhaler)

 Cromolyn (deliver by metered dose inhaler 10–20 minutes before an anticipated provoking stimulus)

   2. When the FEV$_1$ returns to about 50% of normal, patients usually have minimal or no symptoms.
 B. Emergency treatment of asthma (status asthmaticus) includes repetitive administration of a beta-2 agonist by inhalation or injection plus corticosteroids (methylprednisolone 60 to 125 mg IV every 6 hours).
   1. Intubation of the trachea and mechanical support of ventilation may be necessary in the presence of hypercarbia (PaCO$_2$ >50 mmHg) despite aggressive bronchodilator and anti-inflammatory therapy.
   2. In rare circumstances, when life-threatening status asthmaticus persists despite aggressive pharmacologic

therapy, it may be acceptable to consider general anesthesia with a volatile anesthetic in an attempt to produce bronchodilation.

V. MANAGEMENT OF ANESTHESIA

A. **Preoperative Evaluation.** Absence of wheezing or dyspnea suggests that the patient is not experiencing acute exacerbation of asthma.

1. Chest physiotherapy, systemic hydration, appropriate antibiotics, and bronchodilator therapy during the preoperative period will often improve reversible components of asthma, as evidenced by pulmonary function tests (especially FEV_1).

2. Measurement of arterial blood gases before undertaking elective surgery is indicated if there are any questions about the adequacy of ventilation or arterial oxygenation.

B. **Preanesthetic Medication**

1. A preferred drug or combination for use as preanesthetic medication in patients with bronchial asthma has not been established (opioids, anticholinergics and H-2 receptor antagonists may be avoided).

2. Bronchodilator drugs (cromolyn) used in the treatment of asthma should be continued. Supplementation with exogenous corticosteroids may be indicated if adrenal cortex suppression is a possibility.

C. **Induction and maintenance of anesthesia** are designed to depress airway reflexes with anesthetic drugs so as to avoid bronchoconstriction of the hyperreactive airways.

1. **Regional anesthesia** is an attractive choice when the site of operation is superficial or on the extremities, or when avoidance of intubation of the trachea is considered desirable.

2. **General anesthesia** is most often selected for management of the patient with asthma (Table 14-7).

D. **Intraoperative bronchospasm** is usually due to factors other than an acute asthmatic attack (Table 14-8).

1. It is imperative to delay treatment until mechanical obstruction of the breathing circuit and the patient's airway are considered (fiberoptic bronchoscopy is helpful in the diagnosis).

Table 14-7. *Induction and Maintenance of Anesthesia*

Intravenous induction (any currently available drug acceptable; ketamine 1–2 mg•kg^{-1} may produce bronchodilation)

Establish sufficient depth of anesthesia to depress hyperreactive airway reflexes before intubation of the trachea (isoflurane as acceptable as halothane and does not introduce the risk of cardiac dysrhythmias)

Intravenous lidocaine 1–2 mg•kg^{-1} (administer before intubation of the trachea to suppress airway reflexes)

Select muscle relaxants that do not evoke histamine release (atracurium may be avoided; drug-enhanced antagonism is acceptable)

Mechanical ventilation of the lungs (slow inspiratory flow rate provides optimal distribution of ventilation to perfusion; sufficient time for passive exhalation is important to minimize air trapping)

Liberal intravenous fluid replacement

Extubation of trachea while anesthesia is sufficient to suppress hyperreactive airway reflexes (if aspiration a risk, consider lidocaine 1–3 mg•kg^{-1}•h^{-1} IV, to permit toleration of tracheal tube)

Table 14-8. *Differential Diagnosis of Intraoperative Bronchospasm and Wheezing*

Mechanical Obstruction of Tracheal Tube
  Kinking
  Secretions
  Overinflation of cuff

Inadequate Depth of Anesthesia
  Active expiratory efforts
  Decreased functional residual capacity

Endobronchial Intubation

Pulmonary Aspiration

Pulmonary Edema

Pulmonary Embolus

Pneumothorax

Acute Asthmatic Attack

2. Bronchospasm owing to asthma may respond to deepening of anesthesia with a volatile anesthetic, but not to skeletal muscle paralysis.
3. **Albuterol** delivered into the patient's airway by attaching the metered dose inhaler to the anesthesia delivery system via a **T** connector is indicated if bronchospasm persists despite adjustment of the depth of anesthesia.

CHAPTER 15

Restrictive Lung Disease

Restrictive lung disease is characterized by a decrease in total lung capacity and vital capacity (<70 ml·kg^{-1}), most often reflecting an intrinsic disease process that alters the elastic properties of the lung, causing the lungs to stiffen (Fig. 15-1 and Table 15-1) (see Stoelting RK, Dierdorf SF. Restrictive lung disease. In: Anesthesia and Co-Existing Disease. 3rd Ed. New York. Churchill Livingstone, 1993). Expiratory flow rates and the ratio of the forced exhaled volume in 1 second to the forced vital capacity (FEV_1/FVC) is normal, in contrast to patients with chronic obstructive pulmonary disease (see Chapter 13). Patients with restrictive lung disease often complain of dyspnea, reflecting the increased work of breathing in the presence of decreased lung compliance. A rapid, shallow pattern of breathing with an associated decrease in $PaCO_2$ is characteristic, since this minimizes the work of breathing in the presence of decreased lung compliance.

I. PULMONARY EDEMA

A. **Adult respiratory distress syndrome (ARDS)** is characterized by abnormal permeability of pulmonary capillary endothelium, leading to leakage of fluid containing high concentrations of protein into the pulmonary parenchyma and alveoli. Despite improvements in supportive therapy, the mortality rate associated with ARDS over the past 25 years remains unchanged at 60% to 70%. Mortality from ARDS is most often due to multisystem organ failure and systemic hemodynamic instability rather than to lung dysfunction.

1. **Causes.** ARDS is most often associated with shock or sepsis (Table 15-2).
2. **Manifestations** (Table 15-3)
3. **Treatment** (Table 15-4)

B. **Aspiration pneumonitis** reflects destruction of surfactant-producing cells (atelectasis) and damage to pulmonary capillary endothelium (intravascular fluid leaks into the lungs) due to the presence of acidic gastric fluid in the lungs.

1. **Arterial hypoxemia** is the most consistent manifestation of aspiration pneumonitis (Table 15-5).

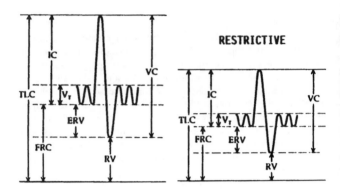

Fig. 15-1. *Lung volumes in restrictive lung disease compared with normal values. In the presence of restrictive lung disease, VC, RV, FRC, and TLC are decreased. TLC, total lung capacity; FRC, functional residual capacity; RV, residual volume; VC, vital capacity; V_T, tidal volume; IC, inspiratory capacity; ERV, expiratory reserve volume.*

Table 15-1. *Causes of Restrictive Lung Disease*

Pulmonary Edema (Acute Intrinsic Restrictive Lung Disease)
    Adult respiratory distress syndrome
    Aspiration
    Neurogenic
    Opioid overdose
    High altitude
    Negative pressure
    Congestive heart failure

Chronic Intrinsic Restrictive Lung Disease
    Sarcoidosis
    Hypersensitive pneumonitis
    Eosinophilic granuloma
    Alveolar proteinosis
    Drug-induced pulmonary fibrosis

Chronic Extrinsic Restrictive Lung Disease
    Obesity

(Continues)

Table 15-1. *Causes of Restrictive Lung Disease* (Continued)

Chronic Extrinsic Restrictive Lung Disease *(cont'd)*
    Ascites
    Pregnancy
    Kyphoscoliosis
    Ankylosing spondylitis
    Deformities of the sternum
    Neuromuscular disorders
        Spinal cord transection
        Guillain-Barré syndrome
        Myasthenia gravis
        Eaton-Lambert syndrome
        Muscular dystrophies
        Pleural fibrosis
        Flail chest

Disorders of the Pleura and Mediastinum
    Pleural effusion
    Pneumothorax
    Mediastinal mass
    Pneumomediastinum

Table 15-2. *Causes of Adult Respiratory Distress Syndrome*

Shock

Sepsis
    Multisystem organ failure
    Acute pancreatitis

Oxygen toxicity

Smoke inhalation

Disseminated intravascular coagulation

Drug-induced

Aspiration

Fat embolism

Pulmonary contusion

Cardiopulmonary bypass

Near-drowning

Table 15-3. *Manifestations of Adult Respiratory Distress Syndrome*

Progressive tachypnea

Arterial hypoxemia despite supplemental oxygen

Hypercarbia

Decreased pulmonary compliance

Lung opacification ("whiteout") on chest radiograph

Pneumonia

Thrombocytopenia

Multisystem organ failure and hemodynamic instability

Table 15-4. *Treatment of Adult Respiratory Distress Syndrome*

Supplemental oxygen

Mechanical ventilation of the lungs if PaO_2 <60 mmHg breathing 50% oxygen

Positive end-expiratory pressure (may adversely decrease venous return)

Diuretics

Inotrope

Table 15-5. *Manifestations of Aspiration Pneumonitis*

Arterial hypoxemia

Tachypnea

Bronchospasm

Pulmonary vascular vasoconstriction

Chest radiograph may remain normal for first 6–12 hours after aspiration

2. **Treatment** of aspiration pneumonitis is delivery of supplemental inspired oxygen and institution of positive end-expiratory pressure. Albuterol by metered dose inhaler may be effective in relieving bronchospasm.

    a. There is no evidence that antibiotics administered pro-phylactically decrease the incidence of pneumonia.

    b. Despite the absence of confirmatory evidence that corticosteroids are beneficial, it is not uncommon for the treatment of aspiration pneumonitis to include the empirical use of pharmacologic doses of these drugs.

C. Neurogenic pulmonary edema reflects massive outpouring of sympathetic nervous system impulses from the injured central nervous system, resulting in generalized vasoconstriction and a shift of blood volume into the pulmonary circulation.

    1. Treatment is normalization of intracranial pressure and support of oxygenation and ventilation.

    2. Digitalis is not indicated in the treatment of neurogenic pulmonary edema as cardiac function is normal.

D. Negative pressure pulmonary edema typically occurs within minutes of the development or relief of acute upper airway obstruction (laryngospasm, epiglottitis). Resolution is typically rapid, and treatment consists of supplemental oxygen and maintenance of a patent upper airway.

II. CHRONIC INTRINSIC RESTRICTIVE DISEASE is characterized by pulmonary fibrosis and loss of pulmonary vasculature leading to dyspnea, pulmonary hypertension, and cor pulmonale (Table 15-1). Pneumothorax is common when pulmonary fibrosis is far advanced.

A. Sarcoidosis is a systemic granulomatous disorder that involves many tissues (liver, spleen, heart), but it has a marked predilection for the thoracic lymph nodes and lungs (fibrosis). Laryngeal sarcoid may occur and interfere with passage of an adult-size tracheal tube. Hypercalcemia is a rare but classic manifestation of sarcoidosis.

    1. Mediastinoscopy is used to provide thoracic lymph node tissue for diagnosis of sarcoidosis.

    2. Corticosteroids are frequently used to treat sarcoidosis associated with restrictive lung disease.

III. CHRONIC EXTRINSIC RESTRICTIVE LUNG DISEASE is most often due to disorders of the thoracic cage that interfere with expansion of the lungs (Table 15-1). The lungs become compressed and lung volumes are decreased.

IV. DISORDERS OF THE PLEURA AND MEDIASTINUM
may contribute to mechanical changes that interfere with optimal expansion of the lungs (Table 15-6).

V. PREOPERATIVE PREPARATION

A. A preoperative history of dyspnea that limits activity and is attributable to restrictive lung disease is an indication for the performance of pulmonary function tests and measurement of arterial blood gases.

1. The most detailed assessment of flow-resistive properties of the airways is obtained by analysis of flow-volume loops (Fig. 15-2).

2. A decrease in vital capacity to <15 ml·kg^{-1} (normal >70 ml·kg^{-1}) or the presence of a resting elevation in the PaCO$_2$ suggests that these patients are at increased risk of the development of exaggerated pulmonary dysfunction during the postoperative period.

3. Eradication of acute pulmonary infection, improvement of sputum clearance, and treatment of cardiac dysfunction are part of the preoperative preparation.

B. Preoperative evaluation of the patient with a **mediastinal mass** includes a chest radiograph, flow-volume loop, computed tomography (evidence of tracheal compression a predictor of airway difficulty during anesthesia), and clinical evaluation of evidence of tracheobronchial compression.

1. The severity of preoperative pulmonary symptoms may bear no relationship to the degree of compromise

---

Table 15-6. *Disorders of the Pleura and Mediastinum*

Pleural effusion

Pneumothorax (severe chest pain and dyspnea; arterial hypoxemia and hypotension likely if tension pneumothorax develops)

Mediastinal mass (superior vena cava syndrome is most often due to cancer; may be evidence of increased intracranial pressure)

Acute mediastinitis

Pneumomediastinum (may follow tracheostomy; treatment rarely necessary)

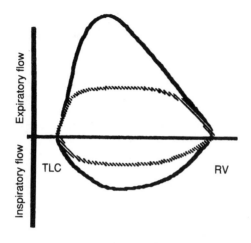

Fig. 15-2. *Flow-volume loop in a normal patient (solid line) and in the presence of an intrathoracic (mediastinal) mass (hatched line). TLC, total lung capacity; RV, residual volume. (From Pullerits J, Holzman R. Anaesthesia for patients with mediastinal masses. Can J Anaesth 1989;36:681–8, with permission.)*

    encountered during anesthesia (supine position may accentuate airway and/or vascular obstruction).

  2. Preoperative radiation should be considered for the patient whose mediastinal tumor is radiation sensitive.

VI. MANAGEMENT OF ANESTHESIA

  A. Restrictive lung disease unrelated to the presence of a mediastinal mass does not influence the choice of drugs used for the induction or maintenance of general anesthesia.

    1. A high index of suspicion for the presence of a pneumothorax and the need to avoid or discontinue nitrous oxide must be maintained.

    2. Regional anesthesia can be considered for peripheral operations, recognizing that high sensory levels of anesthesia may interfere with the patient's ability to maintain acceptable ventilation.

    3. Mechanical ventilation of the lungs during the postoperative period is often required for those patients with

Table 15-7. *Considerations in the Management of Anesthesia in the Presence of a Mediastinal Mass*

External edema associated with superior vena cava syndrome (may be accompanied by intraoral edema; consider gaining intravenous access in the leg)

Awake fiberoptic laryngoscopy (especially in patient who must remain sitting)

Place patient in lateral or prone position should unexpected airway obstruction develop

Spontaneous ventilation and avoidance of skeletal muscle paralysis (may not be possible)

Increased surgical bleeding owing to increased venous pressure

Be prepared to reintubate the trachea postoperatively

Table 15-8. *Diagnostic Techniques*

Fiberoptic bronchoscopy (has replaced rigid scope bronchoscopy; pneumothorax a risk after transbronchial lung biopsies)

Pleuroscopy (alternative to thoracotomy)

Mediastinoscopy (complications include pneumothorax, hemorrhage, venous air embolism, recurrent laryngeal nerve injury, stroke)

impaired pulmonary function documented preoperatively.

B. The method selected for induction of anesthesia and tracheal intubation in the presence of a mediastinal mass depends on the preoperative assessment of the airway (Table 15-7).

VII. DIAGNOSTIC TECHNIQUES (Table 15-8)

CHAPTER 16

Acute Respiratory Failure

Respiratory failure is the inability of the lungs to provide adequate arterial oxygenation with or without acceptable elimination of carbon dioxide (see Stoelting RK, Dierdorf SF. Acute respiratory failure. In: Anesthesia and Co-Existing Disease. 3rd Ed. New York. Churchill-Livingstone, 1993). Fatigue of the muscles of breathing is a principal determinant of acute respiratory failure. Arterial hypoxemia resulting from an intracardiac shunt, anemia, or carbon monoxide poisoning is not considered a cause of acute respiratory failure, since these conditions do not reflect defects in the respiratory system.

I. DIAGNOSIS

    A. Measurement of arterial blood gases (PaO_2, $PaCO_2$) and pH are mandatory in the diagnosis and management of patients with acute respiratory failure (Table 16-1).

    B. Significant desaturation of arterial blood occurs only when the PaO_2 is <60 mmHg, accounting for the common definition of arterial hypoxemia as being a PaO_2 below this level.

    C. Acute respiratory failure is distinguished from chronic respiratory failure on the basis of the relationship of the $PaCO_2$ to pH (normal pH despite an increased PaO_2 reflects compensation by virtue of renal tubular reabsorption of bicarbonate).

II. TREATMENT OF ACUTE RESPIRATORY FAILURE
(Table 16-2)

III. MONITORING OF TREATMENT depends on evaluation of pulmonary gas exchange (arterial and venous blood gases) and cardiac function (cardiac output and cardiac filling pressures). A pulmonary artery catheter is useful in making many of these measurements.

    A. Oxygen Exchange and Arterial Oxygenation. Calculation of the alveolar-to-arterial difference for oxygen ($A-aDO_2$) is useful for evaluating the gas exchange functions of the lungs and for distinguishing between the various mechanisms of arterial hypoxemia (Table 16-3).

Table 16-1. *Diagnosis of Acute Respiratory Failure*

Arterial hypoxemia (PaO_2 <60 mmHg despite supplemental oxygen)

Hypercarbia ($PaCO_2$ >50 mmHg)

Decreased functional residual capacity

Decreased lung compliance

Bilateral diffuse opacification of the lungs on chest radiographs

Table 16-2. *Treatment of Acute Respiratory Failure*

Supplemental oxygen (maintain PaO_2 60–80 mmHg)

Intubation of the trachea

Mechanical support of ventilation (adjust ventilator settings based on arterial blood gases and pH)

Positive-end expiratory pressure (consider when PaO_2 <60 mmHg despite >50% oxygen)

Optimize intravascular fluid volume (guidelines include pulmonary artery occlusion pressure, urine output, and body weight)

Drug-induced diuresis (furosemide)

Inotropic support of cardiac function (offsets adverse effects of positive end-expiratory pressure)

Removal of secretions (bronchoscopy)

Control of infection

Nutritional support (offset skeletal muscle weakness; hyperalimentation may increase metabolic production of carbon dioxide)

Consider prophylactic antacids and/or H-2 antagonists

B. **Carbon Dioxide Elimination.** The adequacy of alveolar ventilation relative to the metabolic production of carbon dioxide is reflected by the $PaCO_2$, whereas the efficacy of carbon dioxide transfer across the alveolar capillary membrane is reflected by the dead space to tidal volume ratio (V_D/V_T) (Table 16-4).

Table 16-3. *Mechanisms of Arterial Hypoxemia*

	PaO_2	$PaCO_2$	$A-aDO_2$	Response to Supplemental Oxygen
Low inspired oxygen concentration (altitude)	D	Normal to D	Normal	Improved
Hypoventilation (drug overdose)	D	I	Normal	Improved
Ventilation-to-perfusion mismatching (COPD, pneumonia)	D	Normal to D	I	Improved
Right-to-left shunt (pulmonary edema)	D	Normal to D	I	Poor to none
Diffusion impairment (pulmonary fibrosis)	D	Normal to D	I	Improved

COPD, chronic obstructive pulmonary disease; D, decrease; I, increase.

Table 16-4. *Mechanisms of Hypercarbia*

	$PaCO_2$	V_D/V_T	$A-aDO_2$
Drug overdose	I	Normal	Normal
Restrictive lung disease (kyphoscoliosis)	I	Normal to I	Normal to I
COPD	I	I	I
Neuromuscular disease	I	Normal to I	Normal to I

COPD, chronic obstructive pulmonary disease; I, increase; D, decrease.

C. **Mixed venous partial pressure of oxygen** ($P\bar{v}O_2$ and the arterial-to-venous difference for oxygen (CaO_2-CvO_2) reflects the overall adequacy of the oxygen transport system (cardiac output) relative to extraction of oxygen by tissues.

1. A decrease in cardiac output that occurs in the presence of unchanged tissue oxygen consumption causes the $P\bar{v}O_2$ to decrease and the CaO_2–CvO_2 to increase.
2. A $P\bar{v}O_2$ <30 mmHg or a CaO_2–CvO_2 >6 ml·dl^{-1} indicates the need to increase cardiac output to facilitate tissue oxygenation.

D. **Accuracy of Blood Gas Measurements**
   1. The recommendation that arterial blood gases should be corrected for differences between the patient's body temperature and the temperature of the measuring electrode (pH-stat management) is based on the known temperature-dependent solubility of oxygen and carbon dioxide in blood.
   2. The argument that PCO_2 and pH do not need to be corrected for temperature (alpha-stat management) is based on the concept that the measured values reflect an unperturbed acid-base status of the patient regardless of the body temperature that existed at the time the sample was drawn.

Table 16-5. *Steps in Cessation of Mechanical Support of Ventilation*

Removal of Ventilator Support
    Vital capacity >15 ml·kg^{-1}
    A-aDO$_2$ <350 mmHg
    PaO$_2$ >60 mmHg (<50% oxygen)
    Normal pH
    Spontaneous breathing rate <20 breaths·min^{-1}
    V$_D$/V$_T$ <0.6
    Co-existing abnormalities (consciousness, cardiac function, electrolyte balance, nutrition)

T Tube Weaning (tachypnea, tachycardia, or deterioration in the level of consciousness is evidence that weaning is premature; addition of continuous positive airway pressure may be useful)

Intermittent Mandatory Ventilation (rate of mandatory breaths guided by pH)

Removal of the Tracheal Tube (must be alert with active laryngeal and cough reflexes)

Elimination of the Need for Supplemental Oxygen (guide by pulse oximetry and measurement of PaO$_2$)

Table 16-6. *Management of Anesthesia for Lung Transplantation*

Strict attention to asepsis

Pulmonary artery catheter

Avoid drug-induced histamine release

Double-lumen endobronchial tube (verify placement by fiberoptic bronchoscopy)

Partial cardiopulmonary bypass may be required

    E. Arterial pH measurement is necessary to detect acidemia (hypoventilation, lactic acidosis) or alkalemia (hyperventilation, hydrogen ion loss) (see Table 21-10).

IV. CESSATION OF MECHANICAL SUPPORT OF VENTILATION. The process of weaning occurs in five steps (Table 16-5).

V. LUNG TRANSPLANTATION

    A. Single lung transplantation is a consideration for patients experiencing end-stage respiratory failure.

    B. Management of anesthesia invokes the principles used in performing anesthesia for pneumonectomy (Table 16-6).

    C. The principal causes of mortality are bronchial dehiscence or respiratory failure owing to infection or rejection.

CHAPTER 17

Diseases of the Nervous System

Perhaps in no other area of anesthesia is the selection of drugs, technique of ventilation of the lungs, and choice of monitors more important than in the care of the patient with a disease involving the central nervous system (CNS) (see Stoelting RK, Dierdorf SF. Diseases of the nervous system. In: Anesthesia and Co-Existing Disease. 3rd Ed. New York. Churchill Livingstone, 1993).

I. INTRACRANIAL TUMORS (Table 17-1)

A. **Diagnosis.** Computed tomography (CT) with contrast enhancement and magnetic resonance imaging have revolutionized the capability of imaging techniques for identifying brain tumors.

B. **Treatment.** Surgery is part of the initial management of virtually all brain tumors, as it establishes the diagnosis and relieves symptoms due to a space-occupying lesion. Radiation therapy is particularly useful for the management of a malignant brain tumor.

C. **Signs and symptoms.** The major mechanism for the production of signs and symptoms by an intracranial tumor is increased intracranial pressure (ICP) (Table 17-2).

D. **Management of anesthesia.** The goals of perioperative anesthesia management are often based on keeping the ICP within a normal range and recognition that autoregulation of cerebral blood flow (CBF) may be impaired.

1. **Pressure-volume compliance curves** reflect changes produced by an expanding intracranial tumor (Fig. 17-1).

   a. Eventually, a point is reached on the curve where even a small increase in intracranial volume produced by the expanding tumor results in a marked increase in the ICP.

   b. It is at this point on the curve that anesthetic drugs and techniques that affect cerebral blood volume can adversely and abruptly increase ICP.

2. **Monitoring ICP** is accomplished by placing a catheter in a cerebral ventricle or a transducer on the surface of the brain.

Table 17-1. *Classification of Brain Tumors*

Primary Brain Tumor
    Histologically Benign
        Meningioma
        Pituitary adenoma
        Astrocytoma
        Acoustic neuroma

    Histologically Malignant
        Glioblastoma
        Medulloblastoma

Metastatic Brain Tumor

Table 17-2. *Signs and Symptoms of Increased Intracranial Pressure*

Evidence of Increased Intracranial Pressure
    Headache
    Nausea and vomiting
    Mental changes
    Disturbances of consciousness
    Hypertension
    Bradycardia
    Midline shift (>0.5 cm) on computed tomography

Seizure

Evidence of Brain Herniation
    Dilated and unreactive pupil
    Contralateral hemiplegia
    Disturbances of consciousness
    Apnea

    a. A normal ICP wave is pulsatile and varies with the cardiac impulse and breathing (normal mean ICP <15 mmHg).
    b. **Plateau wave** is an abrupt and sustained increased in ICP observed during continuous monitoring of ICP (Table 17-3).
  3. Methods to Decrease ICP (Table 17-4)
  4. Determinants of CBF (Fig. 17-2)
    a. The ability of hypocapnia to decrease CBF and ICP is the basis of modern neuroanesthesia.

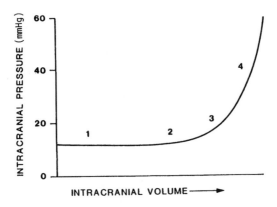

Fig. 17-1. *A pressure-volume compliance curve depicts the impact of increasing intracranial volume on intracranial pressure (ICP). As intracranial volume increases from point 1 to 2, ICP does not increase, since cerebrospinal fluid is shifted from the cranium into the spinal subarachnoid space. A patient with an intracranial tumor but between points 1 and 2 on the curve is unlikely to manifest symptoms of increased ICP. A patient on the rising portion of the curve (3) can no longer compensate for an increase in intracranial volume and ICP begins to increase and is likely to be associated with clinical symptoms. An additional increase in intracranial volume at this point (3), as produced by increased cerebral blood flow during anesthesia, can precipitate an abrupt increase in ICP (4).*

Table 17-3. *Events Identified as Initiating Causes of a Plateau Wave*

Anxiety

Painful stimulation (liberal use of analgesics to avoid pain even in the unresponsive patient)

Induction of anesthesia (establishment of adequate depth of anesthesia before initiating direct laryngoscopy)

---

    b. Autoregulation of CBF may be lost or impaired in the presence of an intracranial tumor or head trauma and the administration of a volatile anesthetic.

    c. Anesthetic drugs. Volatile anesthetics administered during normocapnia in a concentration >0.6 MAC

Table 17-4. *Methods to Decrease Intracranial Pressure*

Posture (avoid head-down position)

Hyperventilation (maintain $PaCO_2$ 25–30 mmHg; effect wanes after about 6 hours)

Cerebrospinal fluid drainage

Hyperosmotic drugs (mannitol 0.25–1 $g \cdot kg^{-1}$ IV)

Diuretics (furosemide 1 $mg \cdot kg^{-1}$ IV)

Corticosteroids (relieve localized cerebral edema that develops around an intracranial tumor)

Barbiturates (consider in presence of acute head injury)

are potent cerebral vasodilators that produce dose-dependent increases in CBF (halothane > enflurane and desflurane > isoflurane) and ICP. The greater decrease in cerebral metabolic oxygen requirements ($CMRO_2$) produced by isoflurane may explain why

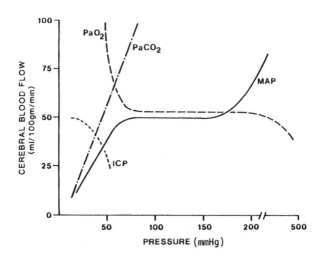

Fig. 17-2. *Schematic depiction of the impact of intracranial pressure (ICP), PaO_2, $PaCO_2$, and mean arterial pressure (MAP) on cerebral blood flow.*

CBF increases are minimal below 1.1 MAC. In hypocapnic patients with supratentorial mass lesions, 1 MAC desflurane, but not isoflurane, produces modest increases in ICP. **Barbiturates and opioids** are cerebral vasoconstrictors that are capable of decreasing CBF with an associated decrease in a previously elevated ICP. Drug-induced **histamine release** could produce cerebral vasodilation and is a consideration in the selection of muscle relaxants, especially succinylcholine and atracurium.

5. **Preoperative evaluation** is directed toward establishing the presence or absence of increased ICP (Table 17-2).
6. **Preoperative medication** using drugs that may depress ventilation and/or level of consciousness must be used sparingly, if at all, in the patient with an intracranial tumor.
7. **Induction of anesthesia** is designed to minimize changes in CBF and ICP both with production of unconsciousness and with intubation of the trachea (Table 17-5).
8. **Maintenance of anesthesia** is often with nitrous oxide plus intravenous supplementation with an opioid and/or barbiturate.
   a. The minimal effects of isoflurane (<0.6 MAC) on

Table 17-5. *Induction of Anesthesia in the Presence of an Intracranial Tumor*

Preoxygenation and consideration of spontaneous hyperventilation

Thiopental (4–6 mg•kg^{-1} IV) (benzodiazepines, etomidate, propofol acceptable alternatives)

Skeletal muscle paralysis (2–3 times ED$_{95}$ of pancuronium, vecuronium, atracurium, or mivacurium; succinylcholine may produce a modest and transient increase in intracranial pressure)

Mechanical hyperventilation of the lungs (PaCO$_2$ 25–30 mmHg)

Intubation of the trachea (consider additional thiopental, opioid, or lidocaine before stimulus; ensure intense paralysis before initiating laryngoscopy)

CBF make this a useful volatile anesthetic in the patient undergoing an intracranial operation.

b. Treatment of hypertension with a direct vasodilator (nitroglycerin, nitroprusside) may increase CBF and ICP despite a simultaneous reduction in systemic blood pressure.

c. Skeletal muscle paralysis is often maintained during intracranial surgery, as unexpected movement can lead to increased ICP or bulging of the brain.

9. **Fluid therapy** is with a hypertonic salt solution (5% glucose in lactated Ringer's solution) at a rate of 1 to 3 $ml \cdot kg^{-1} \cdot h^{-1}$. Glucose-and-water solutions are not recommended, since they are rapidly and equally distributed throughout total body water.

10. **Monitoring** (Table 17-6)

11. **Venous air embolism** is most often associated with neurosurgical procedures in which the operative site is above the level of the heart (veins in cranium are held open by surrounding bone).

a. Detection of venous air embolism is essential (Table 17-7).

b. Treatment (Table 17-8)

12. **Postoperative Management.** Recognition of any adverse effects produced by surgery is facilitated by early dissi-

---

Table 17-6. *Monitoring in the Presence of an Intracranial Tumor*

Intra-arterial blood pressure

Capnography

Intracranial pressure (not routine)

Urine output

Right atrial catheter (pulmonary artery catheter an alternative)

Peripheral nerve stimulator

Doppler transducer (place between the second and third intercostal spaces, just to the right of the sternum)

Electrocardiogram (cardiac dysrhythmias owing to brain stem manipulation)

Table 17-7. *Detection of Venous Air Embolism*

Doppler transducer (most sensitive)

Sudden decrease in end-tidal carbon dioxide concentration

Increase in right atrial and pulmonary artery pressure

Increase in end-tidal nitrogen concentration (may precede changes in end-tidal carbon dioxide concentration or right heart pressure)

Sudden attempts to breath (gasp reflex)

Hypotension, cardiac dysrhythmias, and cyanosis (late signs)

Table 17-8. *Treatment of Venous Air Embolism*

Occlude venous air entry site

Aspirate air via right atrial catheter

Discontinue nitrous oxide

Positive end-expiratory pressure ≤10 cm H_2O

Sympathomimetic and/or inotrope

Beta-2 agonist

pation and/or pharmacologic reversal of the effects of anesthetics and muscle relaxants.

a. It is important to prevent any reaction to the tracheal tube as the patient awakens (consider lidocaine 0.5 to 1.5 mg·kg^{-1} IV).

b. If consciousness was depressed preoperatively or if body temperature decreased to <34°C during surgery, it may be best to delay extubation of the trachea until it can be confirmed that airway reflexes are present. Also, spontaneous ventilation should be sufficient to prevent accumulation of carbon dioxide.

II. CEREBROVASCULAR DISEASE. The major risk factors for the development of cerebrovascular disease are diabetes mellitus and hypertension. Only heart disease and cancer exceed stroke as causes of mortality.

A. **Transient ischemic attack (TIA)** is a temporary focal episode of neurologic dysfunction that develops suddenly and resolves completely within 24 hours. Presumably, this reflects the rapid dissolution of thromboembolism from an atherosclerotic plaque in an extracranial blood vessel.

1. **Carotid artery disease** is a reflection of atheromatous disease (bruit may or may not be detectable).

2. **Vertebrobasilar arterial disease** manifests as symptoms referable to ischemia of the posterior portions of the brain, including the occipital lobes (diplopia) or brain stem (vertigo, ataxia, sudden loss of postural tone in the legs while consciousness is maintained, transient global amnesia).

3. **Medical treatment** of TIA is preferred in the patient with vertebrobasilar arterial disease (long-term administration of an antiplatelet aggregating drug or coumarin anticoagulant).

4. **Surgical treatment** of the patient with a lesion occluding more than 80% of the carotid artery and a history of repeated TIAs is carotid endarterectomy.

   a. **Management of anesthesia** for carotid endarterectomy surgery is intended to **maintain cerebral perfusion pressure and CBF** (Table 17-9). The most critical period is the time of surgical occlusion of the common carotid artery.

   b. **Postoperative Problems** (Table 17-10)

B. **Stroke**

1. **Stroke is categorized** as being due to hemorrhage (subarachnoid hemorrhage from an intracranial aneurysm or intracerebral hemorrhage from rupture of a small artery damaged by hypertension) and ischemia (systemic hypoperfusion, embolism, and thrombosis) (Table 17-11).

2. **Management of anesthesia** for resection of a congenital intracranial aneurysm is designed to prevent dangerous elevations in systemic blood pressure and to facilitate surgical exposure and vascular control of the aneurysm by producing controlled hypotension (Table 17-12).

III. **ACUTE HEAD TRAUMA** most often follows a motor vehicle accident and is frequently associated with other injuries, including cervical spine injury and thoracoabdomi-

Table 17-9. *Management of Anesthesia in the Patient Undergoing Carotid Endarterectomy*

Preoperative Evaluation
    Ischemic heart disease (most likely cause of morbidity and mortality)
    Range of normal blood pressure
    Effects of changes in head position on cerebral function

Choice of Anesthesia
    Regional anesthesia (cervical plexus block; early warning of cerebral dysfunction with arterial cross-clamping)
    General anesthesia (thiopental induction and maintenance with nitrous oxide plus isoflurane or an opioid; consider thiopental just before arterial cross-clamping; goal is maintenance of blood pressure within a normal range for that patient)

Monitor Adequacy of Cerebral Blood Flow
    Electroencephalogram
    Somatosensory evoked potentials
    Stump pressure (influenced by vasoconstricting or vasodilating effects of anesthetic drugs; >60 mmHg probably reflects adequate collateral blood flow)

Table 17-10. *Postoperative Problems Associated With Carotid Endarterectomy*

Hypertension (common during immediate postoperative period, especially in the patient with co-existing hypertension; treat with a vasodilator)

Hypotension

Airway compression due to hematoma at the operative site

Loss of carotid body function

Myocardial infarction

Stroke

Peripheral nerve damage (facial nerve, recurrent laryngeal nerve)

Table 17-11. *Characteristics of Stroke Subtypes*

	Subarachnoid Hemorrhage	Intracerebral Hemorrhage	Systemic Hypoperfusion	Embolism	Thrombosis
Risk factors	Often absent Hypertension Coagulopathy Drugs Trauma	Hypertension Coagulopathy Drugs Trauma	Hypotension Hemorrhage Cardiac arrest	Smoking Ischemic heart disease Peripheral vascular disease Diabetes mellitus White male	Smoking Ischemic heart disease Peripheral vascular disease Diabetes mellitus White male
Onset	Sudden, often during exertion	Gradually progressive	Parallels risk factors	Sudden	Often preceded by a TIA Progressive
Signs and symptoms	Headache Vomiting Transient loss of consciousness	Headache Vomiting Decreased level of consciousness Seizures	Pallor Diaphoresis Hypotension	Headache	Headache
Imaging	CT: hyperdensity (white) MRI	CT: focal hyper-density (white) MRI	CT: low density (black) MRI	CT: low density (black) MRI	CT: low density (black) MRI

CT, computed tomography; MRI, magnetic resonance imaging.

Table 17-12. *Management of Anesthesia for Resection of an Intracranial Aneurysm*

Preoperative Evaluation
Assess mental status (preoperative medication may be indicated to decrease apprehension)
Estimate intracranial pressure

Induction of Anesthesia
Intravenous anesthetic plus a muscle relaxant
Minimize pressor response to intubation of the trachea (see Table 5-7)

Maintenance of Anesthesia
Nitrous oxide plus a volatile anesthetic (attenuates pressor response to noxious stimulation and decreases necessary dose of vasodilator drug required for controlled hypotension)
Management of ventilation, fluid therapy, monitors, increased intracranial pressure (see Table 17-4)

Controlled Hypotension
Nitroprusside (dose seldom >3 $\mu g \cdot kg^{-1} \cdot min^{-1}$; consider use of beta antagonist if reflex tachycardia occurs; tachyphylaxis or metabolic acidosis may reflect onset of cyanide toxicity)
Estimate safe level of blood pressure decrease (guideline is to decrease mean arterial pressure 30–40 mmHg below normal awake level, assuming central venous pressure <10 mmHg and $PaCO_2$ near 35 mmHg)
Monitor blood pressure accurately (transducer at level of circle of Willis)

nal trauma. Initial management includes immobilization of the cervical spine, establishment of a patent upper airway, and protection of the lungs from aspiration of gastric contents.

A. The **Glasgow Coma Scale** provides a reproducible method for assessing the seriousness of brain injury and for following the patient's neurologic status (Table 17-13). Patients with a scale score of 8 are by definition in coma and about 50% of these patients die or remain in a vegetative state.

B. The most useful diagnostic procedure is CT, which should be performed as soon as possible (Table 17-14).

Table 17-13. *Glasgow Coma Scale*

Response	Score
Eye Opening	
Spontaneous	4
To speech	3
To pain	2
Nil	1
Best Motor Response	
Obeys	6
Localizes	5
Withdraws (flexion)	4
Abnormal flexion	3
Extensor response	2
Nil	1
Verbal Response	
Oriented	5
Confused conversation	4
Inappropriate words	3
Incomprehensible sounds	2
Nil	1

Table 17-14. *Diagnostic Value of Computed Tomography in the Patient With Acute Head Trauma*

Epidural Hematoma
  Skull fracture with associated rupture of a meningeal artery
  Initial loss of consciousness followed by lucid interval
  Treatment is burr holes

Subdural Hematoma
  Reflects bleeding from a bridging vein
  Associated head trauma may have seemed trivial, especially in an elderly patient
  Symptoms evolve gradually (headache, drowsiness, lateralizing neurologic signs)
  Treatment is usually surgical evacuation

IV. DEGENERATIVE DISEASES OF THE NERVOUS SYSTEM

A. **Aqueductal stenosis** is caused by congenital narrowing of the cerebral aqueduct that connects the third and fourth ventricles. It leads eventually to obstructive hydrocephalus and symptoms of increased ICP (Table 17-2). Treatment is placement of a ventricular shunt.

B. **Arnold-Chiari malformation** is a herniation of the cerebellum into the cervical spinal canal requiring surgical decompression.

C. **Syringomyelia** is progressive degeneration of the spinal cord (cavitation), leading to sensory and motor (thoracic scoliosis) deficits. The possible absence of protective upper airway reflexes and a hyperkalemic response to succinylcholine are considerations in the management of anesthesia.

D. **Amyotrophic lateral sclerosis** is a degenerative disease of motor cells throughout the CNS and spinal cord, leading to weakness and fasciculations of skeletal muscles. Dysphagia (bulbar involvement) leading to pulmonary aspiration and a hyperkalemic response to succinylcholine are considerations in the management of anesthesia.

E. **Friedreich's ataxia** is characterized by degeneration of the spinocerebellar and pyramidal tracts, often in association with cardiomyopathy and kyphoscoliosis.

F. **Paralysis agitans (Parkinson's disease)** is a degenerative disease of the CNS characterized by loss of dopaminergic fibers (dopamine is an inhibitory neurotransmitter acting on the extrapyramidal motor system) in the basal ganglia of the brain (Table 17-15).

G. **Hallervorden-Spatz disease** is a disorder of basal ganglia characterized by dystonic posturing and scoliosis.

H. **Huntington's chorea** is a premature degenerative disease of the CNS characterized by progressive dementia, pulmonary aspiration, and involuntary skeletal muscle movements.

I. **Spasmodic torticollis** most frequently presents as spasmodic contraction of nuchal muscles that may interfere with maintenance of a patent upper airway in an anesthetized but unparalyzed patient.

J. **Shy-Drager syndrome** is characterized by autonomic nervous system dysfunction (orthostatic hypotension) and degeneration of the CNS and spinal cord. Management of anesthesia includes continuous monitoring of blood pressure and prompt correction of hypotension with infusion of fluids and/or administration of a vasopressor (possible enhanced response to drugs that act by evoking the release of norepinephrine).

Table 17-15. *Characteristics of Paralysis Agitans*

Signs and Symptoms
  Skeletal muscle rigidity
  Resting tremor
  Diaphragmatic spasms
  Mental depression

Treatment (designed to increase the concentration of dopamine in the basal ganglia or decrease the neuronal effects of acetylcholine)
  Levodopa (combine with a decarboxylase inhibitor; side effects reflect dopamine effects on the central nervous system, heart, and gastrointestinal tract)
  Anticholinergic drugs
  Antihistaminic drugs

Management of Anesthesia
  Continue levodopa therapy
  Possibility of blood pressure lability and cardiac dysrhythmias
  Avoid drugs with antidopaminergic effects (droperidol, possibly opioids)

- K. **Congenital insensitivity to pain** with anhidrosis is a rare hereditary disorder that leads to self-mutilation and defective thermoregulation.
- L. **Progressive blindness** due to degenerative diseases of the CNS limited to the optic nerve and retina include Leber's optic atrophy (avoid nitroprusside as vulnerable to cyanide toxicity), retinitis pigmentosa, and Kearns-Sayer syndrome (associated with cardiac conduction abnormalities, including third-degree atrioventricular heart block).
- M. **Alzheimer's disease** is characterized by intellectual deterioration in an adult severe enough to interfere with occupational or social performance. Sedatives and centrally acting anticholinergic drugs are avoided in the management of anesthesia.
- N. **Creutzfeldt-Jakob disease** is a progressively fatal encephalopathy transmissible by an infectious pathogen that is reliably inactivated by steam, ethylene oxide, and sodium hypochlorite.
- O. **Leigh syndrome** is a necrotizing encephalomyelopathy manifesting as hypotonia, seizures, and aspiration in children.

P. Rett syndrome manifests exclusively in females as dementia, autistic behavior, and breathing abnormalities leading to apnea and arterial hypoxemia.

Q. Sotos syndrome is characterized by mental retardation and macrocephaly (airway management difficult), often in association with scoliosis and the likely need for corrective surgery.

R. Multiple sclerosis is characterized by random and multiple sites of demyelination of corticospinal tract neurons in the brain and spinal cord, exclusive of the peripheral nervous system (Table 17-16).

Table 17-16. *Characteristics of Multiple Sclerosis*

Signs and Symptoms (reflect effects of demyelination)
  Visual disturbances
  Ataxia
  Limb paresthesias and weakness
  Spastic paresis of skeletal muscles
  Exacerbations and remissions

Diagnosis
  Somatosensory evoked responses
  Computed tomography
  Immersion in hot water
  Examination of cerebrospinal fluid

Treatment (none curative)
  Corticosteroids
  Avoid stress (surgery)
  Avoid marked environmental temperature changes
  Dantrolene
  Carbamazepine

Management of Anesthesia
  Exacerbation of symptoms may occur independent of anesthetic drugs or technique (spinal anesthesia a questionable selection for this reason)
  Possible hyperkalemic in response to succinylcholine
  Consider need for corticosteroid supplementation
  Prevent increased body temperature postoperatively

S. **Optic neuritis** is eventually associated with evidence of multiple sclerosis in about 50% of patients (Table 17-16).

T. **Transverse myelitis** is inflammation of the spinal cord characterized by rapid ascending weakness of the legs and sensory anesthesia.

U. **Stiff-man syndrome** is characterized by the sudden onset of continuous and intense skeletal muscle rigidity that interferes with ventilation but, unlike tetanus, does not cause trismus.

V. **NEUROPATHIES** may involve cranial or peripheral nerves (Table 17-17). Specific questions during the initial clinical examination can aid in the search for the etiology of the peripheral neuropathy (Table 17-18).

A. **Postoperative neuropathy** is a significant source of anesthetic-related liability claims.

B. **Idiopathic facial paralysis (Bell's palsy)** is characterized by the rapid onset of motor weakness or paralysis (no sensory loss) of facial muscles innervated by the facial nerve.

Table 17-17. *Classification of Neuropathies*

Cranial Mononeuropathies
  Idiopathic facial paralysis (Bell's palsy)
  Trigeminal neuralgia (tic douloureux)
  Glossopharyngeal neuralgia
  Vestibular neuronitis
  Metastatic cancer

Peripheral Entrapment Neuropathies
  Carpal tunnel syndrome
  Ulnar nerve palsy
  Brachial plexus palsy
  Radial nerve palsy
  Meralgia paresthetica
  Femoral nerve palsy
  Peroneal nerve palsy

Peripheral Metabolic Neuropathies
  Alcohol
  Vitamin B_{12} deficiency
  Diabetes mellitus
  Hypothyroidism

(Continues)

Table 17-17. *Classification of Neuropathies* (Continued)

Peripheral Metabolic Neuropathies *(cont'd)*
   Uremia
   Porphyria

Systemic Disease-Related Peripheral Neuropathies
   Cancer
   Sarcoidosis
   Collagen vascular disease
   Acute idiopathic polyneuritis (Guillain-Barré syndrome)

Toxic Peripheral Polyneuropathies
   Drugs
      Sulindac
      Amiodarone
      Hydralazine
      Nitrous oxide
      Disulfiram
      Phenytoin
      Isoniazid
      Cisplatin
      Vincristine
   Industrial agents
   Insecticides
   Heavy metals

Peripheral Hereditary Neuropathies
   Peroneal muscular atrophy (Charcot-Marie-Tooth disease)
   Refsum's disease
   Möbius syndrome

1. **Treatment** is with prednisone and covering of the eye to protect the cornea.
2. Trauma to the facial nerve can reflect stretch injury produced by excessive traction on the angle of the mandible during maintenance of the upper airway in an unconscious patient.
C. **Trigeminal neuralgia (tic douloureux)** is characterized by the sudden onset of brief, but intense, unilateral facial pain triggered by local sensory stimuli applied to the affected side of the face. Medical treatment is with carbamazepine, whereas surgical treatment consists of selective

Table 17-18. *Questions to Determine the Etiology of a Peripheral Neuropathy*

1. Is the disturbance a mononeuropathy or a mononeuropathy multiplex (asymmetric involvement of more than one nerve)? If the answer is yes, the etiology is most likely local entrapment, compression, traction, or ischemia.

2. Is the disturbance a symmetric polyneuropathy? If the answer is yes, the etiology is most likely metabolic, systemic, or toxic (see Table 17-17).

3. Is the neuropathy primarily motor (acute idiopathic polyneuritis, porphyria)?

4. Is the neuropathy primarily sensory (vitamin deficiency)?

5. Is there a family history of neuropathy?

radiofrequency destruction of trigeminal nerve fibers (may be accompanied by systemic hypertension requiring vasodilator therapy) or microsurgical decompression of the trigeminal nerve.

D. Glossopharyngeal neuralgia is characterized by intense pain in the sensory distribution of the nerve (throat, neck, tongue, ear); it is associated with severe bradycardia (sudden death) and seizures.

   1. Treatment is topical anesthesia, administration of carbamazepine, and, in life-threatening situations, intracranial section of the nerve.

   2. Management of Anesthesia (Table 17-19)

E. Carpal tunnel syndrome is the most frequent of the entrapment neuropathies (conduction delay in the median nerve at the wrist) (Fig. 17-3). Surgical decompression is the recommended treatment if conservative measures, such as immobilization and local injection of corticosteroids, do not prove effective.

F. Ulnar nerve palsy is the most common postoperative peripheral neuropathy. The etiology is often not apparent (may appear spontaneously without any relationship to anesthesia and surgery).

   1. The male predominance of perioperative ulnar nerve injury suggests an anatomic predisposition (perhaps

Table 17-19. *Management of Anesthesia in the Patient With Glossopharyngeal Neuralgia*

Anticipate hypovolemia

Consider placement of an artificial transvenous cardiac pacemaker

Topical anesthesia of the oropharynx

Anticholinergic drug promptly available

Postoperative hypertension

Vocal cord paralysis

the depth of the cubital tunnel at the elbow) associated with the male body habitus.

2. The ulnar nerve is probably more susceptible to compression in the cubital tunnel when the elbow is fully flexed and/or the hand is pronated (Fig. 17-4).

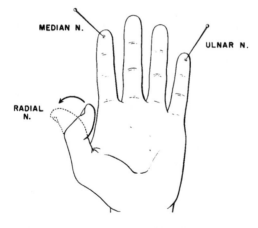

Fig. 17-3. *Schematic diagram for the rapid identification of peripheral nerve injury to the upper extremity. Injury to the musculocutaneous nerve results in loss of biceps function and inability to flex the forearm; injury to the axillary nerve results in loss of deltoid function and inability to abduct the arm. (From McAlpine FS, Seckel BR. Complications of positioning. The peripheral nervous system. In: Martin JT, ed. Positioning in Anesthesia and Surgery. Philadelphia. WB Saunders 1987;303–28, with permission.)*

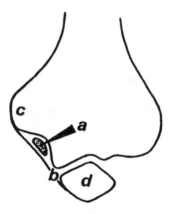

Fig. 17-4. *Schematic depiction of the relationship of the ulnar nerve (a) to the arcuate ligament (b) that extends from the medial epicondyle of the humerus (c) to the olecranon of the ulna (d) at the elbow, forming the roof of the cubital tunnel. Pronation of the forearm rotates the cubital tunnel such that the medial epicondyle and olecranon both rest on the same flat surface and increases the possibility of ulnar nerve compression in the cubital tunnel. Likewise, flexion of the elbow tenses the arcuate ligament and decreases the size of the cubital tunnel. (From Wadsworth TG. The cubital tunnel and the external compression syndrome. Anesth Analg 1974;53:303–8, with permission.)*

  3. Electromyographic studies are indicated when a patient complains of a new postoperative sensory or motor deficit (active denervation potentials do not appear until about 3 weeks after injury).
  G. Brachial plexus palsy may reflect trauma during thoracic surgery, owing to the long course of the nerves of this plexus in the axilla between two points of fixation.
  H. Peroneal nerve palsy reflects compression of the common peroneal nerve at the level of the head of the fibula (Fig. 17-5).
  I. Acute idiopathic polyneuritis (Guillain-Barré syndrome) is characterized by the onset of weakness or paralysis that typically manifests in the legs and spreads cephalad (Table 17-20). Altered function of the autonomic nervous system and the presence of lower motor neuron lesions are the two important considerations for management of anesthesia in these patients (Table 17-21).

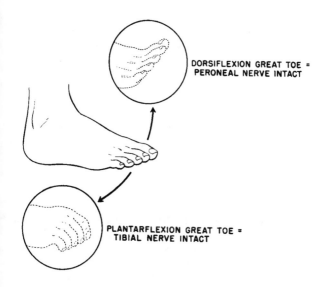

**DORSIFLEXION GREAT TOE =
PERONEAL NERVE INTACT**

**PLANTARFLEXION GREAT TOE =
TIBIAL NERVE INTACT**

Fig. 17-5. *Schematic diagram for the rapid identification of peripheral nerve injury of the lower extremity. Injury to the femoral nerve results in loss of quadriceps function. (From McAlpine FS, Seckel BR. Complications of positioning. The peripheral nervous system. In: Martin JT, ed. Positioning in Anesthesia and Surgery. Philadelphia. WB Saunders 1987;303–28, with permission.)*

Table 17-20. *Characteristics of Acute Idiopathic Polyneuritis*

Ascending flaccid paralysis (lower motor neuron)

Bulbar involvement

Intercostal muscle weakness (monitor vital capacity and arterial blood gases, as may require tracheal intubation and mechanical support of ventilation)

Pharyngeal muscle weakness (aspiration)

Sensory paresthesias and pain

Autonomic nervous system dysfunction (labile blood pressure, cardiac conduction disturbances, sudden death)

Table 17-21. *Management of Anesthesia in the Patient With Acute Idiopathic Polyneuritis*

Hypotension with changes in posture, blood loss, or positive airway pressure (impaired compensatory cardiovascular responses)

Hypertension with noxious stimulation (laryngoscopy)

Exaggerated response to indirect-acting vasopressors

Possible hyperkalemic response to succinylcholine

Anticipate need for postoperative mechanical support of ventilation

VI. **SPINAL CORD TRANSECTION.** Anatomically, the spinal cord is not divided, but the effect physiologically is the same as if it were transected. It is estimated that cervical spine injury occurs in 1.5% to 3% of all major trauma victims. The trauma patient's neck must be promptly immobilized, preferably with a rigid collar. Vertebral injury can occur without cord damage, as the spinal canal is widest in the cervical region. In an alert patient, the absence of neck pain or tenderness virtually eliminates the presence of cervical spine injury.

A. **Pathophysiology** (Table 17-22)

B. **Autonomic hyperreflexia** is a disorder that appears after resolution of spinal shock and in association with cutaneous (surgical incision) or visceral (bladder distension) stimulation below the level of spinal cord transection (Fig. 17-6).

   1. The incidence of autonomic hyperreflexia depends on the level of spinal cord transection (85% when above T10 and unlikely when below T10). Surgery, however, is a particularly potent stimulus to the development of autonomic hyperreflexia. Even patients with no previous history of this response may be at risk during operative procedures.

   2. **Signs and Symptoms** (Table 17-23)

C. **Management of anesthesia** in a patient with transection of the spinal cord is largely determined by the duration of the injury (Table 17-24). Regardless of the duration of spinal cord transection, the institution of preoperative

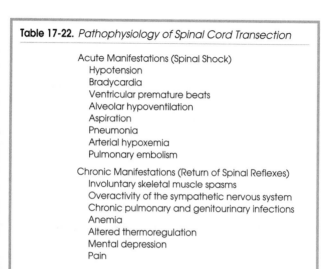

Table 17-22. *Pathophysiology of Spinal Cord Transection*

Acute Manifestations (Spinal Shock)
Hypotension
Bradycardia
Ventricular premature beats
Alveolar hypoventilation
Aspiration
Pneumonia
Arterial hypoxemia
Pulmonary embolism

Chronic Manifestations (Return of Spinal Reflexes)
Involuntary skeletal muscle spasms
Overactivity of the sympathetic nervous system
Chronic pulmonary and genitourinary infections
Anemia
Altered thermoregulation
Mental depression
Pain

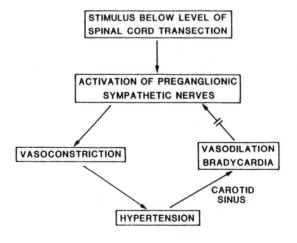

Fig. 17-6. *Schematic diagram of the sequence of events associated with clinical manifestations of autonomic hyperreflexia. Impulses that produce vasodilation cannot reach the neurologically isolated portion of the spinal cord, such that vasoconstriction and hypertension persist.*

Table 17-23. *Signs and Symptoms of Autonomic Hyperreflexia*

Hypertension and bradycardia

Vasodilation above the level of spinal cord transection (nasal stuffiness)

Headache

Subarachnoid hemorrhage

Seizures

Cardiac dysrhythmias

Acute left ventricular failure (pulmonary edema)

Table 17-24. *Management of Anesthesia in the Presence of Spinal Cord Transection*

Acute Spinal Cord Transection
  Avoid extension of the head during direct laryngoscopy, if cervical spine injury is present or a possibility
  Absence of compensatory cardiovascular responses manifested during posture change, blood loss, or positive airway pressure
  Guard against hypothermia
  Need for muscle relaxant dictated by operative site (pancuronium useful; succinylcholine safe within first 24 hours after acute injury)

Chronic Spinal Cord Transection
  Prevent autonomic hyperreflexia (general versus spinal anesthesia; nitroprusside promptly available)
  Exclusive use of nondepolarizing muscle relaxants

hydration is helpful in preventing hypotension during induction and maintenance of anesthesia.

VII. CEREBRAL PROTECTION AND RESUSCITATION

A. **Cardiac arrest** produces **global cerebral ischemia** (irreversible injury may require >4 minutes to develop). It may be followed within 15 to 90 minutes after resuscitation by profound cerebral hypoperfusion owing to increased cerebral small vessel vascular resistance.

1. Historically, management of a patient who fails to awaken after cardiac arrest has included hypothermia (only method to depress $CMRO_2$ requirements below that needed for normal cellular function), hyperventilation of the lungs (does not improve outcome in absence of increased ICP), and large doses of corticosteroids (unproved efficacy).

2. **Barbiturates** do not improve outcome after global cerebral ischemia produced by a cardiac arrest. This is predictable because the electroencephalogram (EEG) becomes flat within 20 to 30 seconds after cardiac arrest, and subsequent administration of a barbiturate would not be expected to further decrease $CMRO_2$ of cells. In contrast to global ischemia, incomplete ischemia **(focal cerebral ischemia)** with maintenance of electrical activity on the EEG is likely to be associated with improved neurologic outcome when a barbiturate is administered to produce metabolic suppression.

3. **Postanoxic encephalopathy.** The prognosis for acceptable neurologic recovery is about 1% for patients who remain comatose 24 hours after resuscitation from a cardiac arrest and in whom two of three reflexes (pupillary, corneal, oculovestibular) are absent.

4. **Brain death** is suggested by the presence of coma, absence of evidence of brain stem function (apnea), isoelectric EEG, and absence of cerebral circulation.

B. **Stroke.** On the basis of current animal data, production of barbiturate coma in stroke patients cannot be recommended.

C. **Head Injury.** The greatest success in cerebral protection and resuscitation has been with patients who have experienced head injury.

1. **Barbiturates** are recommended when ICP remains elevated despite traditional therapy (Table 17-4). The goal of barbiturate therapy is to maintain ICP <20 mmHg without the occurrence of plateau waves. The presence of an isoelectric EEG confirms the presence of maximum drug-induced depression of $CMRO_2$.

2. Hypotension produced by barbiturate therapy may interfere with the maintenance of an adequate cere-

bral perfusion pressure and may require inotropic support of cardiac output.

VIII. **EPILEPSY** (seizure disorder) is estimated to occur in 2% to 5% of the population at some time during their life (Table 17-25).

   A. **Pathophysiology.** A seizure results from the excessive discharge of an aggregate of neurons that depolarize in a synchronous fashion (may remain localized or spread).

   B. **Treatment** of chronic epilepsy is ideally with a single nonsedating drug (often valproic acid), usually selected on the basis of the classification of the seizure disorder (Table 17-25).

   C. **Grand mal seizure** (status epilepticus) is a life-threatening medical emergency as adequate ventilation and oxygenation is not possible without appropriate treatment (Table 17-26).

   D. **Management of Anesthesia** (Table 17-27)

Table 17-25. *Classification of Adult Seizure Disorders*

Type	Clinical Features	Effective Drugs	Half-time (h)	Therapeutic Blood Level ($\mu g \cdot ml^{-1}$)
Partial (Focal)				
Simple partial	Focal motor or sensory disturban-ces (Jack-sonian epilep-sy) Conscious-ness not impaired	Valproic acid	12	50–100
		Carbama-zepine	12	4–10
		Phenytoin	24	10–20
Complex partial	Bizarre behavior and impaired conscious-ness Auras prominent	As for simple partial seizures		

(Continues)

Table 17-25. *Classification of Adult Seizure Disorders* (Continued)

Type	Clinical Features	Effective Drugs	Half-time (h)	Therapeutic Blood Level ($\mu g \cdot ml^{-1}$)
Generalized Absence	Brief loss of consciousness, staring, little or no motor activity	Valproic acid Ethosuximide	55	50–100
Myoclonic	Isolated clonic jerks often evoked by a sensory stimulus	Valproic acid		
Continual Status epilepticus	Continual seizure activity	Diazepam Phenytoin Carbamazepine Valproic acid	24	10–20

Table 17-26. *Treatment of a Grand Mal Seizure*

Establish patent upper airway

Administer oxygen

Diazepam (2 mg·min^{-1} IV), until seizure stops or reaches 20 mg

Phenytoin (50 mg·min^{-1}) (prevents recurrence as effect of diazepam wanes)

General anesthesia and muscle relaxant (only in patients who do not respond to conventional treatment; muscle relaxant alone does not interfere with continuous firing of neurons)

Table 17-27. *Management of Anesthesia in a Patient With a Seizure Disorder*

Consider effects of anticonvulsant therapy (sedation, enzyme induction)

Selection of drugs for anesthesia may be influenced by effects on central nervous system electrical activity

  Methohexital (may activate epileptic foci)

  Ketamine (unpredictable effects)

  Enflurane (spike and wave activity)

  Atracurium (laudanosine a stimulant)

Drugs that do not predispose to seizure activity

  Thiobarbiturates

  Benzodiazepines

  Opioids

  Isoflurane

  Halothane

  Desflurane

IX. SYNCOPE is a sudden transient loss of consciousness followed by spontaneous recovery (must be differentiated from seizures). The most common causes of syncope are vasovagal reactions, orthostatic hypotension, drug-induced, and cardiac disease.

X. HEADACHE is usually benign. During the postoperative period, it may reflect perioperative caffeine withdrawal (Table 17-28).

Table 17-28. *Characteristics of Headaches Encountered During the Perioperative Period*

Migraine Headache

  Visual blurring

  Nausea and vomiting

  Traditional explanation is cerebral vasoconstriction, followed by vasodilation (abnormal serotonergic transmission may be more likely)

  Treatment is ergonovine or methysergide (selective agonist of serotonin receptors may also be effective)

(Continues)

Table 17-28. *Characteristics of Headaches Encountered During the Perioperative Period* (Continued)

Migraine Headache *(cont'd)*
No known anesthetic hazards (consider possible drug interactions with ergot preparations)

Cluster Headache (Histamine Cephalgia)
Excruciating unilateral temple or malar pain (visual disturbances; ptosis and miosis may occur)
Treatment is often unsatisfactory (ergot preparations; intranasal lidocaine)

Increased Intracranial Pressure (see Table 17-2)

Benign Intracranial Hypertension (Pseudotumor Cerebri)
ICP >20 mmHg in absence of a focal intracranial lesion
Often an obese female
Treatment is daily lumbar puncture to remove 20–40 ml of fluid (may add acetazolamide and dexamethasone; lumboperitoneal shunt in resistant patients)
Management of anesthesia as if an intracranial tumor is present (spinal anesthesia may be therapeutic but, if shunt present, may be ineffective as local anesthetic is lost)

XI. HERNIATION OF AN INTERVERTEBRAL DISC
(Table 17-29)

XII. SLEEP DISORDERS

A. **Insomnia** is the most common sleep disorder. It occurs especially in females and elderly patients.
   1. About 10% to 15% of patients with chronic insomnia have an underlying problem of substance abuse, especially alcohol.
   2. Benzodiazepines because of their efficacy and safety are the drugs of choice for the treatment of insomnia.
B. **Narcolepsy** is an uncontrollable urge to sleep. It may be accompanied by sudden loss of postural tone (cataplexy).
C. **Sleep apnea syndrome** (cessation of airflow at the mouth for >10 seconds) can reflect loss of CNS drive to maintain

---

Table 17-29. *Herniation of an Intervertebral Disc*

Cervical Disc Disease
  Lateral protrusion of a cervical disc occurs at C5-C6 (neck pain radiates down arm to thumb) or C6-C7 (pain in scapula to middle and index fingers)

  Treatment is traction, followed by surgical decompression if necessary

Cervical Spondylosis
  Narrowing of spinal canal and compression of the spinal cord by osteophytes
  Neck and shoulder pain accompanied by sensory loss and skeletal muscle wasting

Lumbar Disc Disease
  Low back pain estimated to occur in almost 80% of adults at some time
  Computed tomography diagnostic of disc protrusion at L4-L5 or L5-S1 (pain radiates down lateral aspect of the thigh)

  Treatment is bed rest (2 days as effective as longer periods), steroid epidural, laminectomy if neurologic symptoms persist

---

ventilation (central sleep apnea) or mechanical upper airway obstruction (obstructive sleep apnea).

1. **Signs and Symptoms** (Table 17-30)
2. **Treatment** (Table 17-31)

Table 17-30. *Signs and Symptoms of Sleep Apnea Syndrome*

Signs	Symptoms
Obesity	Insomnia
Hypertension	Intense snoring
Arterial hypoxemia	Thrashing during sleep
Hypercarbia	Morning headache
Polycythemia	Daytime somnolence
Cor pulmonale	Intellectual deterioration

Table 17-31. *Treatment of Sleep Apnea Syndrome*

Obstructive Sleep Apnea
  Correction of nasal obstruction
  Weight loss
  Avoidance of alcohol and sedatives
  Continuous positive nasal airway pressure
  Tracheostomy
  Uvulopalatopharyngoplasty

Central Sleep Apnea
  Avoidance of alcohol and sedatives
  Acetazolamide
  Electrophrenic pacing

3. **Management of anesthesia** must consider the likely **exquisite sensitivity to drugs that depress ventilation** and the possibility of **airway obstruction** with the induction of anesthesia.
   a. Prolonged mechanical ventilation of the lungs may be required postoperatively.
   b. Full return of consciousness should be ensured before extubation of the trachea after uvulopalatopharyngoplasty.
   c. Postoperative pain relief poses an additional risk. Neuraxial opioids have been recommended so as to minimize systemic effects of these drugs on ventilation.

XIII. ABNORMAL PATTERNS OF VENTILATION
(Table 17-32)

XIV. ACUTE MOUNTAIN SICKNESS is most likely due to cerebral edema with ascent to altitude >3660 m. Prompt descent and oxygen therapy are the principal treatments.

XV. EPISTAXIS originating from the anterior nasal chamber (most often from a blood vessel in the mucous membrane of the nasal septum) often stops spontaneously or with application of conservative measures (cold, pressure). Spontaneous bleeding from posterior aspects of the nasal chamber is likely to be arterial and associated with hyper-

Table 17-32. *Abnormal Patterns of Ventilation*

	Pattern	Site of Lesion
Ataxic (Biot's breathing)	Unpredictable sequence of breaths varying in rate and tidal volume	Medulla
Apneustic breathing	Repetitive gasps with prolonged pauses at full inspiration	Pons
Cheyne-Stokes	Cyclic crescendo-decrescendo tidal volume pattern interrupted by apnea	Cerebral hemispheres Congestive heart failure
Central neurogenic hyperventilation	Hypocarbia	Cerebral thrombosis or embolism
Posthyperventilation apnea	Awake apnea after moderate decreases in the $PaCO_2$	Frontal lobes

tension; it requires treatment with sedation and placement of a postnasal pack (Foley catheter in an emergency). Systemic antibiotics are indicated when a postnasal pack is placed. Obstruction of the nasal airway may also result in arterial hypoxemia, particularly in an elderly debilitated patient.

XVI. MIDDLE EAR COMPLICATIONS RELATED TO USE OF NITROUS OXIDE

A. Narrowing of the eustachian tubes by acute inflammation or the presence of scar tissue, as is likely after an adenoidectomy, impairs the ability of the middle ear to vent passively any pressure increase produced by nitrous oxide.

   1. Tympanic membrane rupture may accompany nitrous oxide-induced increases in middle ear pressure.

   2. Disruption of previous middle ear reconstructive surgery may manifest as recurrence of hearing loss on awakening from anesthesia.

   3. Administration of nitrous oxide during tympanoplasty may result in displacement of a freshly placed graft.

B. Absorption of nitrous oxide after discontinuation of the administration of this drug may result in transient hearing loss or serous otitis reflecting negative pressure in the middle ear.

XVII. GLAUCOMA is characterized by increased intraocular pressure. It requires interventions designed to decrease this pressure by decreasing resistance to outflow of aqueous humor (pilocarpine, timolol) or by reducing the rate of formation of aqueous humor (acetazolamide).

A. Management of Anesthesia (Table 17-33)
B. Postoperatively, the glaucoma patient is observed for evidence of an acute attack (dilated irregular pupil, pain in and around the eye). By contrast, the patient with a corneal abrasion will complain of pain only in the eye.

XVIII. CATARACT EXTRACTION may be performed using a retrobulbar block or under general anesthesia (Table 17-34).

XIX. OCULAR TRAUMA characterized by a penetrating eye injury balances protection of the airway against the hazard of producing an increase in intraocular pressure and the potential extrusion of intraocular contents. The use of succinylcholine in this situation is controversial.

XX. GLOMUS JUGULARE TUMORS (Chemodectomas)

Table 17-33. *Management of Anesthesia in the Glaucoma Patient*

Continue drug therapy (maintain miosis)

Anticholinergic drug acceptable in preoperative medication

Avoid prolonged increases in intraocular pressure
    Succinylcholine (peak in 4–6 minutes, transient)
    Hypercarbia
    Increased central venous pressure

Consider drug interactions
    Echothiophate prolongs succinylcholine
    Timolol may result in bradycardia

Table 17-34. *Management of Anesthesia for Cataract Extraction*

> Retrobulbar Block (passage of local anesthetic into the subarachnoid space can lead to apnea)
>
> General Anesthesia
> - Likely to be elderly with co-existing medical diseases
> - Immobile patient is mandatory when eye is open (consider skeletal muscle paralysis)
> - Short- or intermediate-acting muscle relaxant an alternative to succinylcholine
> - Hypocarbia and head-up tilt will likely decrease intraocular pressure
> - Consider early tracheal extubation
> - Minimize incidence of vomiting during the postoperative period

A. **Signs and symptoms** are related to the vascularity of the tumor (bruit) and invasion of surrounding structures (hearing loss, dysphagia, aspiration, upper airway obstruction, hydrocephalus). It is common for a glomus jugulare tumor to invade the internal jugular vein.

B. **Management of Anesthesia** (Table 17-35)

Table 17-35. *Management of Anesthesia for Excision of a Glomus Jugulare Tumor*

> Preoperative evidence of aspiration or increased intracranial pressure
>
> Invasive monitoring (avoid cannulation of a central vein invaded by tumor)
>
> Hypothermia
>
> Controlled hypotension
>
> Venous air embolism (sudden death may be attributable to this event)
>
> Need to identify facial nerve may influence selection of muscle relaxant

Table 17-36. *Signs and Symptoms of Neurofibromatosis*

Café au lait spots

Neurofibromas
    Cutaneous
    Neural
    Vascular

Intracranial tumor

Spinal cord tumor

Pseudarthrosis

Kyphoscoliosis

Short stature

Cancer

Endocrine dysfunction

Learning disability

Seizures

Congenital heart disease
    Pulmonic stenosis

XXI. CAROTID SINUS SYNDROME is caused by exaggeration of normal activity of baroreceptors (bradycardia, hypotension) in response to mechanical stimulation. Infiltration of lidocaine around the carotid sinus may improve hemodynamic stability.

XXII. NEUROFIBROMATOSIS

A. Signs and Symptoms (Table 17-36)

B. Management of anesthesia must consider the multiple clinical features of this disease (possible presence of pheochromocytoma, increased ICP, upper airway obstruction).

CHAPTER 18

Diseases of the Liver and Biliary Tract

Diseases of the liver and biliary tract can be categorized as parenchymal liver disease (acute and chronic hepatitis, cirrhosis of the liver) and cholestasis with or without obstruction of the extra-hepatic biliary pathway (see Stoelting RK, Dierdorf SF. Diseases of the liver and biliary tract. In: Anesthesia and Co-Existing Disease. 3rd Ed. New York. Churchill Livingstone, 1993).

I. PHYSIOLOGIC FUNCTIONS OF THE LIVER
(Table 18-1)

II. HEPATIC BLOOD FLOW
   A. The liver receives a dual afferent blood supply from the hepatic artery (25% of the total flow but up to 50% of the hepatic oxygen requirements) and vein. Total hepatic blood flow is approximately 1450 ml·min^{-1} or about 30% of cardiac output.
   B. Causes of decreases in hepatic blood flow include volatile anesthetics, surgical stimulation, intra-abdominal operations, and fibrotic constriction characteristic of hepatic cirrhosis.

III. LIVER FUNCTION TESTS are useful to appreciate the presence of liver disease preoperatively and to facilitate the differential diagnosis of postoperative liver dysfunction (Table 18-2).
   A. Liver function tests are rarely specific. Considerable hepatic damage may be present before these tests are altered.
   B. Postoperatively, the magnitude of hepatic dysfunction, as reflected by liver function tests, is exaggerated by operations close to the liver, independent of the anesthetic drugs selected.
   C. The liver is the sole site of synthesis of **albumin.** Significant liver disease is implied by a plasma albumin concentration <2.5 g·dl^{-1}.

IV. DIFFERENTIAL DIAGNOSIS OF POSTOPERATIVE HEPATIC DYSFUNCTION (Table 18-2)

Table 18-1. *Physiologic Functions of the Liver*

Glucose homeostasis

Fat metabolism

Protein synthesis
  Drug binding
  Coagulation
  Hydrolysis of ester linkages

Drug and hormone metabolism

Bilirubin formation and excretion

Table 18-2. *Liver Function Tests and Differential Diagnosis*

Hepatic Dysfunction	Bilirubin	Transaminase Enzymes	Alkaline Phosphatase	Causes
Prehepatic	Increased unconjugated fraction	Normal	Normal	Hemolysis Hematoma resorption Bilirubin overload from whole blood
Intrahepatic (hepato-cellular)	Increased conjugated fraction	Markedly increased	Normal to slightly increased	Viral Drugs Sepsis Hypoxemia Cirrhosis
Posthepatic (cholestatic)	Increased conjugated fraction	Normal to slightly increased	Markedly increased	Stones Sepsis

A. Causes of postoperative hepatic dysfunction are probably multifactorial. Maintenance of hepatic oxygen delivery relative to demand during exposure to anesthetics is important, as **hepatocyte hypoxia** is likely to be important in the etiology of postoperative hepatic dysfunction.

B. When postoperative hepatic dysfunction occurs, specific steps should be taken in search of a cause before assuming, without supporting evidence, that the anesthetic drugs are the responsible hepatotoxins (Table 18-3).

V. ACUTE HEPATITIS

A. **Viral hepatitis** (Table 18-4)
1. **Signs and Symptoms** (Table 18-5)
2. **Epidemiology.** Special features permit differentiation of the various forms of hepatitis (Table 18-4).
    a. **Hepatitis C virus** causes most, if not all, cases of post-transfusion hepatitis.
    b. **Epstein-Barr virus and cytomegalovirus** are infrequent causes of acute hepatitis in adults.

Table 18-3. *Specific Steps in Search of Cause of Postoperative Hepatic Dysfunction*

1. Review all drugs administered
2. Check for sources of sepsis
3. Evaluate bilirubin load (a single unit of whole blood contains 250 mg bilirubin)
4. Rule out occult hematomas
5. Rule out hemolysis
6. Review perioperative records for etiologic factors (hypotension, hypoxemia, hypoventilation, hypovolemia)
7. Consider extrahepatic abnormalities (congestive heart failure, pulmonary embolism, renal failure)

Table 18-4. *Characteristic Features of Viral Hepatitis*

	Type A	Type B	Type C	Type D
Transmission	Fecal-oral, contaminated shellfish	Percutaneous, venereal	Percutaneous	Percutaneous
Incubation period (d)	20–37	60–110	35–70	60–110

(Continues)

Table 18-4. *Characteristic Features of Viral Hepatitis* (Continued)

	Type A	Type B	Type C	Type D
Results of serum antigen and antibody tests	IgM early and IgG during convalescence	HBsAg and anti-HBc early and persist in carriers	Anti-HVC in 6 months	Anti-HVD late and may be short-lived
Immunity	45% have antibodies	5–15% have anti-HBs	Unknown	Protected if immune to type B
Course	Does not progress to chronic liver disease	Chronic liver disease develops in 1–10%	Chronic liver disease develops in 10–40%	Co-exists with type B
Prevention	Pooled gamma globulin	Hepatitis B vaccine, hepatitis B immunoglobulin	Unknown	Unknown
Mortality	≤0.2%	0.3–1.5%	Unknown	2–20%

Table 18-5. *Incidence of Symptoms in Acute Viral Hepatitis*

Symptoms	Patients (%)
Dark urine	94
Fatigue	91
Anorexia	90
Nausea	87
Fever	76
Emesis	71
Headache	70
Abdominal discomfort	65
Light-colored stools	52
Pruritus	42

VI. DRUG-INDUCED HEPATITIS represents rare idiosyncratic drug reactions that are unpredictable, not dose dependent, and often indistinguishable histologically from viral hepatitis.

A. **Anesthetic Drugs** (Table 18-6)

1. Development of an enzyme-linked immunosorbent assay for detection of antibodies evoked by acetylation of liver proteins would help detect those rare patients who have become sensitized by prior exposure to halothane. They are thus at presumed increased risk of subsequent exposure to other volatile anesthetics that are also metabolized to trifluoroacetic acid.

2. Considering the magnitude of metabolism, it is predictable that the incidence of anesthetic-induced hepatitis owing to an immune-mediated mechanism would be greatest after halothane, intermediate with enflurane, and lowest after administration of isoflurane and desflurane.

Table 18-6. *Anesthetic Drugs and Drug-Induced Hepatitis*

Halothane (two types of hepatotoxicity)
    Nonspecific drug effect (most likely reflects changes in hepatic blood flow that impair hepatocyte oxygenation; characterized by transient increases in aminotransferase concentrations; mild and self-limited)
    Halothane hepatitis (most likely an immune-mediated response as evidenced by prior exposure and formation of antibodies that react with neoantigens formed by the interaction of an oxidative trifluoroacetyl halide metabolite of halothane with hepatic microsomal proteins; genetic susceptibility likely; may be fatal)

Enflurane and Isoflurane
    Nonspecific drug effect (as described for halothane)
    Hepatitis (an oxidative halide metabolite of both anesthetics is capable of acetylating the same liver proteins rendered antigenic by the trifluoroacetyl halide metabolite of halothane; cross-sensitivity exists between halogenated anesthetics)

VII. CHRONIC HEPATITIS (Table 18-7)

A. A genetic predisposition to the development of chronic active hepatitis is suggested by the frequency of specific histocompatibility antigens.

B. Potentially hepatotoxic drugs should be avoided and drugs that are metabolized in the liver titrated to effect.

VIII. CIRRHOSIS OF THE LIVER is a sequela of a variety of chronic diseases (most often excess alcohol intake), characterized by scarring of the liver parenchyma that leads to resistance to flow through the portal vein (portal hypertension). As a result, the proportion of hepatic flow delivered via the portal vein is decreased and the contribution to total hepatic blood flow from the hepatic artery is increased. Therefore, decreases in systemic perfusion pressure or arterial oxygenation, as may occur during the perioperative period, are more likely to jeopardize the adequacy of hepatic blood flow and delivery of oxygen to the liver in patients with cirrhosis, as compared with normal patients.

A. Types of Cirrhosis (Table 18-8)

B. Complications of Cirrhosis (Table 18-9)

IX. MANAGEMENT OF ANESTHESIA IN THE PATIENT WITH HEPATIC CIRRHOSIS. It is estimated that 5% to 10% of all patients with cirrhosis of the liver undergo surgery during the last 2 years of life.

Table 18-7. *Differentiating Features in Chronic Hepatitis*

Features	Chronic Active Hepatitis	Chronic Persistent Hepatitis
Jaundice	Common	Rare
Aminotransferases	Markedly increased	Mildly increased
Bilirubin	Increased	Normal
Gamma globulin	Increased	Normal
Prothrombin time	Prolonged	Normal
Albumin	Decreased	Normal
HBsAg (incidence)	10–20%	10–20%

Table 18-8. *Types of Cirrhosis*

Alcoholic hepatitis (concomitant malnutrition is likely; weight loss offset by ascitic fluid; hepatosplenomegaly)

Postnecrotic cirrhosis (females; primary liver cell carcinoma may develop)

Primary biliary cirrhosis (pruritus, prolonged prothrombin time, and osteoporosis)

Hemochromatosis (diabetes mellitus, congestive heart failure, and primary liver cell carcinoma may develop)

Wilson's disease (hepatolenticular degeneration) (esophageal varices, hemolytic anemia, and skeletal muscle rigidity)

Alpha-1-antitrypsin globulin deficiency

Jejunoileal bypass

Table 18-9. *Complications of Hepatic Cirrhosis*

Portal vein hypertension

Varices

Ascites

Hyperdynamic circulation

Cardiomyopathy

Anemia

Coagulopathy

Arterial hypoxemia

Hepatorenal syndrome

Hypoglycemia

Duodenal ulcer

Gallstones

Impaired immune defense

Hepatic encephalopathy

Hepatic cancer

Preoperative criteria may correlate with surgical risk and with postoperative outcome of patients with cirrhosis of the liver who are undergoing major surgery (Table 18-10).

A. **Acute hepatic failure.** Only surgery designed to correct a life-threatening situation should be considered.

   1. Preoperative correction of coagulation abnormalities with fresh frozen plasma may be indicated.

   2. Provision of exogenous glucose is important.

B. **Sober Alcoholic Patient** (Table 18-11)

C. **Intoxicated Alcoholic Patient**

   1. In contrast to the chronic but sober alcoholic, the acutely intoxicated patient requires less anesthetic, as there is an additive depressant effect between alcohol and anesthetics.

   2. Intoxicated patients may be more vulnerable to regurgitation of gastric contents, as alcohol slows gastric emptying and decreases the tone of the lower esophageal sphincter.

   3. Surgical bleeding may reflect alcohol-induced interference with platelet aggregation.

X. IDIOPATHIC HYPERBILIRUBINEMIA (Table 18-12)

XI. ORTHOTOPIC LIVER TRANSPLANTATION

A. Preoperative disturbances include arterial hypoxemia, anemia, thrombocytopenia, disseminated intravascular

Table 18-10. *Prediction of Surgical Risk Based on Preoperative Evaluation*

	Minimal	Modest	Marked
Bilirubin (mg·dl⁻¹)	<2	2–3	>3
Albumin (g·dl⁻¹)	>3.5	3–3.5	<3
Prothrombin time (seconds prolonged)	1–4	4–6	>6
Encephalopathy	None	Moderate	Severe
Nutrition	Excellent	Good	Poor
Ascites	None	Moderate	Marked

Table 18-11. *Management of Anesthesia in the Sober Alcoholic Patient*

Isoflurane may be associated with the best maintenance of hepatic blood flow and hepatocyte oxygenation.

Injected anesthetics are useful, but a cumulative effect is possible.

Postoperative liver dysfunction is likely to be exaggerated, regardless of drug selected.

Alcohol-induced cardiomyopathy is possible.

Anticipate resistance to effects of anesthetic drugs.

Consider impact of hepatic elimination when selecting nondepolarizing muscle relaxants.

Provision of exogenous glucose may be important.

Likelihood of postoperative renal failure is increased in the presence of jaundice.

Avoid esophageal instrumentation in the patient with known esophageal varices.

Table 18-12. *Idiopathic Hyperbilirubinemia*

Gilbert syndrome (defect is decreased bilirubin uptake by hepatocytes; present in varying degrees in 5–10% of the population)

Crigler-Najjar syndrome (decreased or absent glucuronyl transferase enzyme)

Dubin-Johnson syndrome

Benign postoperative intrahepatic cholestasis

coagulation, hypokalemia, hypocalcemia, cardiac failure, and encephalopathy.

B. Management of Anesthesia

1. The need to clamp the abdominal aorta and suprahepatic inferior vena cava dictates placement of arterial and venous catheters above the diaphragm.

2. Massive blood and fluid requirements dictate the use of cell-saver devices and administration of calcium.

   3. Decreased venous return when the inferior vena cava is clamped (consider veno-venous bypass) may require use of inotropes or sympathomimetics.
   4. Metabolic acidosis and derangements of blood glucose concentration are predictable.
   5. Selection of injected drugs must consider the role of the liver in their elimination.
      a. Ketamine is useful for induction of anesthesia and isoflurane with or without opioids may be selected for maintenance of anesthesia.
      b. Nitrous oxide is usually not administered because of the risk of air embolism at the time of revascularization of the liver.

XII. **DISEASES OF THE BILIARY TRACT.** An estimated 15 to 20 million adults in the United States have biliary tract disease, manifesting as gallstones.

   A. **Acute cholecystitis** is almost always due to obstruction of the cystic duct by gallstones, resulting in the abrupt onset of severe midepigastric pain that must be distinguished from other possible causes (Table 18-13).
   B. **Chronic Cholelithiasis and Choledocholithiasis**
      1. Patients who experience repeated attacks of acute cholecystitis eventually develop a fibrotic gallbladder that is not capable of contracting to expel bile.
      2. Acute common bile duct obstruction by a gallstone produces symptoms similar to those of acute cholecystitis.
   C. **Elimination of gallstones** is by surgical removal (open

---

Table 18-13. *Differential Diagnosis of Acute Cholecystitis*

Acute viral hepatitis

Alcoholic hepatitis

Penetrating peptic ulcer

Appendicitis

Pyelonephritis

Right lower lobe pneumonia

Pancreatitis

Myocardial infarction

Table 18-14. *Management of Anesthesia for Cholecystectomy*

Laparoscopic Cholecystectomy
    Impaired venous return owing to abdominal insufflation
    Risk of venous carbon dioxide embolism
    Intraoperative decompression of the stomach
    Observation for accidental injury to abdominal structures
    Loss of hemostasis may require prompt laparotomy

Open Cholecystectomy
    Opioids may cause spasm of the choleduchoduodenal sphincter (many still use opioids as incidence of opioid-induced sphincter spasm is considered to be low)
    Postoperative pain is intense (neuraxial opioids contribute to early ambulation)

cholecystectomy, laparoscopic laser cholecystectomy) or dissolution (dissolve with chemicals or shock wave lithotripsy).
  D. Management of Anesthesia (Table 18-14)

CHAPTER 19

Diseases of the Gastrointestinal System

The principal function of the gastrointestinal tract is to provide the body with a continual supply of water, nutrients, and electrolytes (see Stoelting RK, Dierdorf SF. Diseases of the gastrointestinal system. In: Anesthesia and Co-Existing Disease. 3rd Ed. New York. Churchill Livingstone, 1993).

I. **ESOPHAGEAL DISEASES.** Dysphagia is the classic symptom produced at some stage in all disorders of the esophagus (Table 19-1).

A. **Duodenal ulcer disease** is most common in males. The cause is not known. Critically ill patients may be at increased risk of the development of peptic ulcer disease with bleeding (antacids and/or H-2 antagonists may be administered to maintain gastric fluid pH >3.5).

1. **Signs and symptoms.** The typical complaint is aching pain in the midepigastrum. Complications of duodenal ulcer disease typically manifest as bleeding, gastrointestinal obstruction, and perforation.

2. **Treatment.** Oral antacids are the mainstay of duodenal ulcer therapy with H-2 receptor antagonists, sucralfate, and anticholinergics serving as alternative therapies (Table 19-2). Surgical treatment (vagotomy and pyloroplasty) is used less often than in the past, reflecting the effectiveness of medical therapy. Continuous nasogastric suction is the initial treatment of gastric outlet obstruction or posterior perforation into the pancreas.

B. **Gastrinoma** is a tumor that stimulates parietal cells to secrete enormous amounts of hydrochloric acid (Zollinger-Ellison syndrome is present when intractable pain and ulcers develop).

1. Other endocrine neoplasias are present in about one-fourth of patients (see Table 22-19).

2. **Management of anesthesia** for surgical excision of a gastrinoma must consider the likelihood of a large gastric fluid volume at induction of anesthesia. Depletion

Table 19-1. *Disorders of the Esophagus*

Diffuse esophageal spasm (mimics angina pectoris and responds to nitroglycerin)

Chronic peptic esophagitis (heartburn) (occurs in one-third of adults, reflecting reflux of acidic gastric fluid into the esophagus due to decreased tone of the lower esophageal sphincter; treatment is oral antacids; exclude pneumonia preoperatively; routine H-2 antagonist prophylaxis controversial)

Hiatus hernia (can be identified in about 30% of patients undergoing an upper gastrointestinal radiographic examination; routine H-2 antagonist prophylaxis is controversial as reflux during general anesthesia is unlikely in the absence of upper airway obstruction or reaction to the tracheal tube)

Achalasia (dilated esophagus due to aperistalsis and hypertonia of the lower esophageal sphincter)

Collagen vascular disease

Esophagitis due to drugs

Esophagitis and stricture due to caustic chemicals

Esophageal infections (*Candida albicans* in immunosuppressed patients)

Esophageal diverticula (may predispose to aspiration)

Table 19-2. *Side Effects of H-2 Antagonists*

Decreased hepatic blood flow
Inhibition of P-450 enzyme system
Mental confusion
Leukopenia and thrombocytopenia
Interstitial nephritis
Hepatitis
Polymyositis
Bradycardia and hypotension
Gynecomastia

of intravascular fluid volume and electrolyte imbalance (hypokalemia and metabolic alkalosis) may accompany profuse watery diarrhea.

C. **Gastric ulcer,** in contrast to the more common duodenal ulcer, is associated with normal gastric acid secretion or even hypochlorhydria.

II. IRRITABLE BOWEL SYNDROME is characterized by generalized bowel discomfort often with associated symptoms of vasomotor instability (tachycardia, hyperventilation, fatigue, headache).

III. INFLAMMATORY BOWEL DISEASE (Table 19-3)

A. **Ulcerative colitis** is an inflammatory disease of the colonic mucosa that affects primarily the rectum and distal colon (Table 19-4). **Treatment** may include corticosteroids, electrolyte and intravascular fluid volume replacement, and proctocolectomy.

B. **Crohn's disease** is characterized by ileal and colonic involvement (granulomatous ileocolitis) or disease restricted to the small intestine (regional enteritis) or colon (Table 19-5).

C. **Pseudomembranous enterocolitis** is often associated with antibiotic therapy or intestinal ischemia manifested as dehydration, hypotension, and metabolic acidosis.

D. **Management of anesthesia** for surgical treatment of inflammatory bowel disease requires preoperative evalua-

Table 19-3. *Comparative Features of Ulcerative Colitis and Crohn's Disease*

Feature	Ulcerative Colitis	Crohn's Disease
Acute toxicity	Common	Rare
Stools	Bloody, watery	Watery
Perirectal involvement	Occurs in 10–20% but usually self-limiting	Rectocutaneous fistulas in 50%
Extracolonic complications	Common	Common
Carcinoma of colon	5% after 10 years	1% but not related to extent or duration of the disease
Treatment	Proctocolectomy is curative	Recurrence likely despite surgical resection

tion of intravascular fluid volume and electrolyte status, as well as assessment of both colonic and extracolonic complications (Tables 19-4 and 19-5).

1. Underlying liver disease may influence the choice of volatile anesthetic and muscle relaxant.
2. In the presence of bowel distension, administration of nitrous oxide may be limited or avoided.
3. The need to provide additional corticosteroids during the perioperative period may be a consideration.

IV. **CARCINOID TUMORS** are the most common neoplasms of the small intestine (can mimic acute appendicitis). Diagnosis is supported by increased urinary excretion

Table 19-4. *Complications Associated with Ulcerative Colitis*

Complication	Incidence (%)
Colonic	
Toxic megacolon	1–3
Intestinal perforation	3
Carcinoma of the colon	2.5–30
Hemorrhage	4
Stricture	10
Extracolonic	
Erythema nodosum	3
Iritis	5–10
Ankylosing arthritis	5–10
Fatty liver infiltration	40
Pericholangitis	30–50
Cirrhosis of the liver	3

Table 19-5. *Complications Associated With Crohn's Disease*

Rectal fissures and perirectal abscesses
Intra-abdominal fistulas (often the reason for surgery)
Arthritis
Iritis
Renal stones
Gallstones
Anemia
Hypoalbuminemia (may require hyperalimentation)

of 5-hydroxyindoleacetic acid, which is the degradation product of serotonin.

A. **Carcinoid syndrome** is present when vasoactive substances (serotonin, kallikreins, histamine) released from cells of carcinoid tumors result in clinical symptoms (Table 19-6).

    1. Overall, carcinoid syndrome develops in about 5% of patients with carcinoid tumor.

    2. **Management of Anesthesia** (Table 19-7)

Table 19-6. *Signs and Symptoms of the Carcinoid Syndrome*

Bronchoconstriction–asthma

Tricuspid regurgitation and/or pulmonic stenosis

Premature atrial beats and supraventricular tachydys-rhythmias

Episodic cutaneous flushing or cyanosis

Venous telangiectasia

Chronic abdominal pain and diarrhea

Hepatomegaly

Hyperglycemia

Decreased plasma albumin concentrations

Table 19-7. *Management of Anesthesia in the Patient With a Carcinoid Tumor*

Preoperative preparation with a drug that blocks effects of released vasoactive substances (octreotide, somatostatin)

Hypotension may stimulate release of vasoactive substances (avoid deep anesthesia, drug-induced histamine release, and peripheral sympathetic nervous system blockade)

Avoid activation of sympathetic nervous system, since catecholamines are known to activate kallikreins (ketamine an unlikely selection)

V. DISEASES OF THE PANCREAS

A. **Acute pancreatitis** is manifested as an elevated plasma amylase concentration in a patient experiencing intense midepigastric pain (Table 19-8). Treatment of acute pancreatitis is with nasogastric suction, fluid and electrolyte repletion, and opioids for analgesia.

B. **Chronic pancreatitis** characteristically presents in emaciated males who are chronic alcoholics. Mild diabetes mellitus is common; fatty liver infiltration is likely to be present.

VI. GASTROINTESTINAL BLEEDING (Table 19-9)

A. Most acute gastrointestinal bleeding is self-limited, such

Table 19-8. *Signs and Symptoms of Acute Pancreatitis*

Predisposing conditions (alcohol abuse, gallstones, blunt abdominal trauma, penetrating peptic ulcer, cardiopulmonary bypass)

Increased bilirubin and alkaline phosphatase concentrations

Hypotension and hypovolemia (renal failure a risk)

Hypocalcemia

Pleural effusion

Intestinal ileus

Table 19-9. *Causes of Upper Gastrointestinal Bleeding*

Cause	Incidence (%)
Duodenal ulcer	27
Gastritis	23
Varices	14
Esophagitis	13
Gastric ulcer	8
Mallory-Weiss tear	7
Bowel infarction	3
Idiopathic	5

that 80% or more of patients treated with conservative medical management cease bleeding within 24 to 48 hours.
   B. Hypotension associated with massive gastrointestinal hemorrhage may result in myocardial infarction, renal failure, and hepatic centrilobular necrosis.

VII. DISEASES PRODUCING MALABSORPTION AND MALDIGESTION (Tables 19-10 and 19-11)

VIII. DIVERTICULOSIS AND DIVERTICULITIS (Table 19-12)

IX. GASTROINTESTINAL POLYPS

   A. **Colonic polyps** are the most prevalent gastrointestinal polyps and may be premalignant.
   B. **Familial polyposis coli** is an autosomal dominant trait treated by total colectomy, as the incidence of malignant degeneration, if untreated, is nearly 100%.

Table 19-10. *Diseases Associated With Malabsorption or Maldigestion*

Malabsorption (Small Intestine Defects)	Maldigestion (Pancreatic Defects)
Celiac sprue	Chronic pancreatitis
Tropical sprue	Bile salt deficiency syndrome
Diabetes mellitus	Postgastrectomy steatorrhea
Resection of the ileum	
Ischemia of the small intestine	
Radiation enteritis	
Regional enteritis	
Amyloidosis	
Systemic mastocytosis	
Acquired immunodeficiency syndrome	

Table 19-11. *Differences Between Malabsorption (Small Intestine Disease) and Maldigestion (Pancreatic Disease)*

	Malabsorption	Maldigestion
Weight loss	Marked	Mild to absent
Vitamin deficiency (A, B, E, K, B_{12})	Common	Rare
Anemia	Common (usually megaloblastic)	Rare (unless associated with alcoholism)
Hypoalbuminemia	Common	Rare
Hypomagnesemia	Common	Rare
Steatorrhea	Moderate (<35 g·d^{-1})	Marked (40–80 g·d^{-1})

Table 19-12. *Signs and Symptoms of Diverticulosis and Diverticulitis*

Diverticulosis
Multiple outpouchings of the colonic mucosa
Bleeding may require colectomy

Diverticulitis
Develops in about 1% of patients who have diverticulosis
Abdominal pain, bacteremia, diarrhea leading to hypokalemia and hypovolemia

Acute Appendicitis
Occurs in about 7% of U.S. population
Signs and symptoms related to stage of the disease (incidence of perforation increases rapidly after 72 hours) and location of the appendix (retrocecal)
Ultrasonography a useful diagnostic test (value of leukocytosis and fever is controversial)
Differential diagnosis includes acute salpingitis, tubal pregnancy, ovarian cysts, mesenteric adenitis, perforated duodenal ulcer

CHAPTER 20

Renal Disease

The possibility of impaired renal function during the intraoperative and postoperative period should be considered in those with co-existing renal disease (often elderly patients) and in otherwise healthy patients undergoing major operations (see Stoelting RK, Dierdorf SF. Renal disease. In: Anesthesia and Co-Existing Disease. 3rd Ed. New York. Churchill Livingstone, 1993).

I. FUNCTIONAL ANATOMY OF THE KIDNEYS
(Fig. 20-1)

A. **Endocrine Function.** In addition to serving as target organs for various hormones (parathormone, aldosterone, antidiuretic hormone), the kidneys are involved in both the metabolism (insulin) and secretion (renin) of regulatory substances.

B. **Glomerular filtration rate (GFR)** is predictably decreased (normal 125 ml·min^{-1}) by hypotension, hemorrhage, or dehydration.

C. **Renal blood flow** is autoregulated and is equivalent to 20% to 25% of the resting cardiac output.

II. TESTS FOR EVALUATION OF RENAL FUNCTION (Table 20-1).
Renal function tests are insensitive measurements (at least one-half of normal renal function may be lost before tests of GFR become abnormal). **Trends are more useful than isolated measurements** in evaluating renal function.

III. EFFECTS OF ANESTHETIC DRUGS ON RENAL FUNCTION

A. Anesthetic drugs predictably are associated with decreases in GFR, renal blood flow, and urine output that most likely reflect anesthetic-produced decreases in cardiac output and blood pressure. These changes are attenuated by preoperative hydration.

B. **Direct nephrotoxicity** secondary to fluoride resulting from metabolism of fluorinated volatile anesthetics (enflurane and sevoflurane > isoflurane) may result in polyuria that leads to dehydration, hypernatremia, and increased plasma osmolarity.

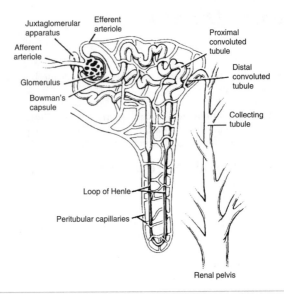

Fig. 20-1. *The functional unit of the kidneys is the nephron, which consists of the glomerulus and the renal tubule.*

Table 20-1. *Tests Used for Evaluation of Renal Function*

Glomerular Filtration Rate (GFR)
   Blood urea nitrogen (10–20 mg·dl^{-1}; influenced by
      diet but when >50 mg·dl^{-1} can assume renal dys-
      function; congestive heart failure the most com-
      mon nonrenal cause of an increase)
   Plasma creatinine (0.7–1.5 mg·dl^{-1}; not influenced
      by diet but does parallel skeletal muscle mass)
   Creatinine clearance (110–150 ml·min^{-1}; most reli-
      able clinical estimate of GFR)

Renal Tubular Function
   Urine concentrating ability
   Sodium excretion
   Proteinuria
   Hematuria
   Urine sediment
   Urine volume

IV. CHRONIC RENAL FAILURE

A. Despite different causes (diabetic nephropathy, chronic glomerulonephritis, pyelonephritis), the common denominator present in patients in whom chronic renal failure develops is progressive and irreversible loss of functioning nephrons with an associated decrease in GFR.

   1. Renal reserve is decreased, but patients remain asymptomatic when >40% of the nephrons continue to function.

   2. Loss of >90% of functioning nephrons results in uremia and the need for dialysis.

B. **Characteristic Changes** (Table 20-2)

C. **Management of Anesthesia.** The most important observation is an assessment of whether the disease is stable, progressing, or improving, as confirmed by **monitoring the plasma concentration of creatinine.** Preservation of renal function intraoperatively depends on **maintaining an ade-**

Table 20-2. *Changes Characteristic of Chronic Renal Failure*

Chronic Anemia
    Increased cardiac output
    Oxyhemoglobin dissociation curve shifted to the right

Coagulopathy
    Platelet dysfunction
    Systemic heparinization

Altered Hydration and Electrolyte Balance
    Unpredictable intravascular fluid volume
    Hyperkalemia
    Hypermagnesemia
    Hypocalcemia

Metabolic Acidosis

Systemic Hypertension
    Congestive heart failure
    Attenuated sympathetic nervous system activity due to therapy with antihypertensive drugs

Increased Susceptibility to Infection
    Decreased activity of phagocytes
    Immunosuppressant drugs

quate intravascular fluid volume and minimizing cardiovascular depression.

1. **Preoperative evaluation** includes consideration of concomitant drug therapy and evaluation of those changes
considered characteristic of chronic renal failure
(Table 20-2). In addition to patients with known preoperative renal dysfunction, it is important to recognize others who are at high risk of perioperative renal
failure, even in the absence of co-existing renal disease.
   a. Diabetes mellitus is often present.
   b. Estimates of blood volume status are based on body
weight before and after hemodialysis, consideration
of vital signs (orthostatic hypotension, heart rate),
and measurement of atrial filling pressures.
   c. Preoperative medication is individualized, remem-
bering the possibility of unexpected sensitivity to
central nervous system depressant drugs.
   d. Uremia may be associated with slowing of gastric
emptying.

2. **Induction of anesthesia** and intubation of the trachea
can be safely accomplished with intravenous drugs
(propofol, etomidate, barbiturates, midazolam) plus
succinylcholine (mivacurium or atracurium an alternative). Regardless of blood volume status, these patients
often respond to induction of anesthesia as if they are
hypovolemic.

3. **Maintenance of anesthesia** is often achieved with
nitrous oxide combined with isoflurane, halothane,
desflurane, or a short-acting opioid.
   a. A potent volatile anesthetic is useful in controlling
intraoperative hypertension and in decreasing the
dose of muscle relaxant needed for adequate surgical relaxation.
   b. When hypertension does not respond to an adjustment in the depth of anesthesia, it may be appropriate to administer a vasodilator such as hydralazine
or nitroprusside.

4. **Regional anesthesia** such as brachial plexus block is
useful for the placement of a vascular shunt necessary
for chronic hemodialysis. Adequacy of coagulation is
considered before proceeding with regional anesthesia.

5. **Muscle Relaxants.** Clearance mechanisms influence the drug selected with mivacurium and atracurium and, to a somewhat lesser extent, vecuronium, as the most useful nondepolarizing muscle relaxants for administration of patients with severe renal disease. **Recurarization** after drug-enhanced reversal of neuromuscular blockade is unlikely because plasma clearance of anticholinesterase drugs will be delayed as long as, if not longer than, the nondepolarizing muscle relaxants.

6. **Fluid management and urine output.** Preoperative hydration with a balanced salt solution (10 to 20 ml·kg^{-1}), followed by administration of 3 to 5 ml·kg^{-1}·h^{-1} intraoperatively may be recommended to maintain urine output >0.5 ml·kg^{-1}·h^{-1}.

   a. Stimulation of urine output with an osmotic (mannitol) or tubular (furosemide) diuretic in the absence of adequate intravascular fluid volume replacement is not recommended.

   b. In the absence of renal function, replacement of insensible fluid losses is with 5% glucose in water.

7. **Monitoring** may include measurement of cardiac filling pressures to facilitate fluid replacement and to recognize the need for inotropic support.

8. **Postoperative Management** (Table 20-3)

V. PERIOPERATIVE OLIGURIA

A. Acute perioperative oliguria (<0.5 ml·kg^{-1}·h^{-1}) must be treated promptly. The responsible causes, if prolonged, may lead to acute renal failure with a mortality >50% (Table 20-4).

B. The usual differential diagnosis is between prerenal (undamaged renal tubules conserve sodium in an attempt

---

Table 20-3. *Postoperative Management of the Patient With Chronic Renal Failure*

Recurarization

Hypertension

Possible increased sensitivity to opioids

Cardiac dysrhythmias

Table 20-4. *Causes of Perioperative Oliguria*

Prerenal (Decreased Renal Blood Flow)
  Hypovolemia
  Decreased cardiac output

Renal (Acute Tubular Necrosis)
  Renal ischemia due to prerenal causes
  Nephrotoxic drugs
  Release of hemoglobin or myoglobin

Postrenal
  Bilateral ureteral obstruction
  Extravasation due to bladder rupture

---

to restore intravascular fluid volume) and renal (damaged renal tubules limited in ability to conserve sodium) causes (Table 20-5).

C. The most common cause of acute renal failure is prolonged (30 to 60 minutes) renal hypoperfusion, owing most often to hypovolemia.

D. **Treatment**
   1. Aggressive and early treatment of perioperative oliguria is most important for those patients at increased risk of the development of acute renal failure (Table 20-6).
   2. Occurrence of transient oliguria during an elective operation in a young patient without co-existing renal disease does not require the same aggressive treatment as does oliguria in an elderly patient with co-existing renal disease (Fig. 20-2).

VI. PRIMARY DISEASES OF THE KIDNEYS
(Table 20-7)

Table 20-5. *Differential Diagnosis of Perioperative Oliguria*

	Prerenal	Renal
Urine sodium (mEq·L^{-1})	<40	>40
Urine osmolarity (mOsm·L^{-1})	>400	250–300
Urine osmolarity/plasma osmolarity	>1.8	<1.1

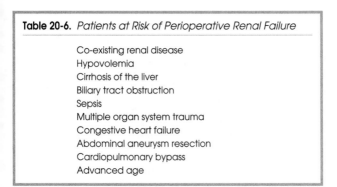

Table 20-6. *Patients at Risk of Perioperative Renal Failure*

Co-existing renal disease
Hypovolemia
Cirrhosis of the liver
Biliary tract obstruction
Sepsis
Multiple organ system trauma
Congestive heart failure
Abdominal aneurysm resection
Cardiopulmonary bypass
Advanced age

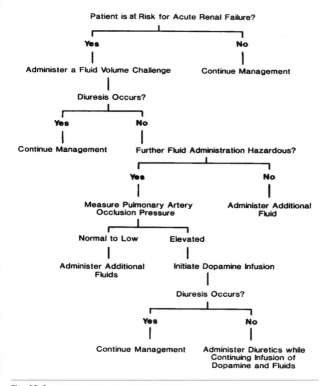

Fig. 20-2. *Treatment of perioperative oliguria.*

Table 20-7. *Primary Diseases of the Kidneys*

Glomerulonephritis (most common cause of end-stage renal failure in adults)

  Acute nephritic syndrome (follows streptococcal infection in children; proteinuria and hypertension)

  Goodpasture syndrome (pulmonary hemorrhage and glomerulonephritis)

  Nephrotic syndrome (hypoalbuminemia leads to edema and ascites; thromboembolic episodes; treatment is corticosteroids)

  Interstitial nephritis (allergic reaction to drugs)

Polycystic Renal Disease

Fanconi Syndrome (polyuria, metabolic acidosis, hypokalemia)

Bartter Syndrome (hypokalemic, hypochloremic metabolic alkalosis; overproduction of prostaglandins)

Renal Hypertension (renal disease the most frequent cause of secondary hypertension)

Uric Acid Nephropathy (most likely in patients with myeloproliferative diseases being treated with cancer chemotherapeutic drugs)

Hepatorenal Syndrome (decompensated cirrhosis of the liver in association with decreased glomerular filtration rate)

VII. NEPHROLITHIASIS

  A. Although the pathogenesis of renal stones is poorly understood, known predisposing factors are recognized for the five major types of stones (Table 20-8).
  B. **Treatment.** Extracorporeal shock wave lithotripsy is a noninvasive treatment of renal stones that requires some form of anesthesia (Table 20-9).

VIII. BENIGN PROSTATIC HYPERTROPHY (BPH)

  A. Definitive treatment of BPH is transurethral resection of the prostate (TURP).
  1. The intravascular absorption of fluids used to distend the bladder during the surgical procedure may pro-

Table 20-8. *Composition and Characteristics of Renal Stones*

Type of Stone	Incidence (%)	Radiographic Appearance	Etiology
Calcium oxalate	65	Opaque	Primary hyperparathyroidism Idiopathic hypercalciuria Hyperoxaluria Hyperuricosuria
Magnesium ammonium phosphate (struvite)	20	Opaque	Alkaline urine (usually due to chronic bacterial infection)
Calcium phosphate	7.5	Opaque	Renal tubular acidosis
Uric acid	5	Lucent	Acid urine, gout Hyperuricosuria
Cystine	1.5	Opaque	Cystinuria

Table 20-9. *Management of Anesthesia for Extracorporeal Shock Wave Lithotripsy*

Immobilization important, as any movement may displace the stone from the focus site

Mechanical ventilation of the lungs using a slow breathing rate

Sensory level to T6 if regional anesthesia selected

Effects of water immersion
  Hydrostatic pressure on thorax and abdomen
  Diuresis
  Hypothermia
  Electrical hazard

Hypotension when removed from bath

Cardiac dysrhythmias during delivery of shock waves

duce cardiovascular and central nervous system manifestations, known as the TURP syndrome (Table 20-10).

Table 20-10. *Manifestations of the TURP Syndrome*

Cardiovascular	Central Nervous System
Hypertension	Restlessness
Increased central venous pressure	Confusion
Bradycardia	Nausea
Myocardial ischemia	Visual disturbances
Shock	Seizures
	Coma

2. The intravascular absorption of large volumes of electrolyte-free fluid leads to **dilutional hyponatremia** (Table 20-11).
3. It is estimated that 10 to 30 ml of irrigating fluid is absorbed into the patient's circulation for every minute of operating time (reason to attempt to keep resection time <60 minutes).

B. **Management of Anesthesia** (Table 20-12)

IX. **RENAL TRANSPLANTATION** is considered for selected patients with end-stage renal disease (diabetes mellitus, hypertension) who are on an established program of chronic hemodialysis.

A. **Management of Anesthesia** (Table 20-13)
B. **Complications** (Table 20-14)

Table 20-11. *Manifestations of Acute Hyponatremia*

Serum Sodium $(mEq \cdot L^{-1})$	Electrocardiogram	Central Nervous System
120	Possible widening of QRS	Restlessness Confusion
115	Widened QRS Elevated ST segment	Nausea Somnolence
110	Ventricular tachycardia Ventricular fibrillation	Seizures Coma

Table 20-12. *Management of Anesthesia for TURP*

Spinal Anesthesia (T10 sensory level)
   Early detection of excessive intravascular absorption of irrigation fluid
   Early detection of bladder perforation
   Postoperative analgesia if morphine added to local anesthetic solution
General Anesthesia (desirable approach when patients cannot cooperate)
Monitor for Signs of Hemodilution
   Serum sodium concentration
   Serum osmolarity
   Hematocrit
   Ethanol in exhaled breath if using a tagged irrigation fluid
Assess Blood Loss (estimate at 15 ml•g^{-1} of tissue resected)

Table 20-13. *Management of Anesthesia for Renal Transplantation*

Preoperative hemodialysis
Blood glucose concentration if patient diabetic
Regional anesthesia (eliminates need for tracheal intubation and muscle relaxants; risks are hypovolemia and coagulopathy)
General anesthesia (isoflurane and atracurium common selections)
Fluid management (5% glucose with 0.45% sodium chloride)
Consider mannitol to facilitate urine formation by the newly transplanted kidney

Table 20-14. *Complications After Renal Transplantation*

Cardiac arrest (sudden hyperkalemia with release of the vascular clamp)
Acute immunologic rejection (may be accompanied by disseminated intravascular coagulation)
Hematoma
Delayed signs of rejection (fever, oliguria)
Lymphoma

CHAPTER 21

Water, Electrolyte, and Acid-Base Disturbances

Alterations of water and electrolyte content and distribution as well as acid-base disturbances can produce multiple organ system dysfunction during the perioperative period (Table 21-1) (see Stoelting RK, Dierdorf SF. Water, electrolyte, and acid-base disturbances. In: Anesthesia and Co-Existing Disease. 3rd Ed. New York. Churchill Livingstone, 1993). Often the manifestations of these disturbances are related more to the rate of change and less to the absolute change.

I. DISTRIBUTION OF BODY WATER

  A. **Total body water content** is greatest at birth and subsequently decreases with increasing age (Fig. 21-1).

  B. Total body water content is categorized as **intracellular** or **extracellular** (interstitial and intravascular), according to the location of water relative to cell membranes (Fig. 21-2 Table 21-2).

II. DISTRIBUTION OF ELECTROLYTES differs greatly among the fluid compartments for body water (Table 21-3).

III. ELECTROPHYSIOLOGY OF CELLS is dependent on an unequal distribution of ions across cell membranes (excess potassium inside and sodium outside cells) that creates an electrochemical difference with the interior of the cell being negative relative to the exterior (Fig. 21-3).

IV. TOTAL BODY WATER EXCESS results in **hyponatremia** (sodium concentration <135 mEq·L^{-1}) and **peripheral edema.**

  A. **Signs and symptoms** of total body water excess depend on the absolute plasma sodium concentration and its rate of decline (Table 21-4).

  B. **Treatment** of excess body water is to reduce the water content of the brain by administering hypertonic saline, mannitol, or furosemide.

  C. **Inappropriate secretion of antidiuretic hormone (ADH)**

Table 21-1. *Etiology of Water, Electrolyte, and Acid-Base Disturbances During the Perioperative Period*

Disease States
    Endocrinopathies
    Nephropathies
    Gastroenteropathies

Drug Therapy
    Diuretics
    Corticosteroids

Nasogastric Suction

Surgery
    Transurethral resection of the prostate
    Translocation of fluid due to tissue trauma
    Resection of portions of the gastrointestinal tract

Management of Anesthesia
    Intravenous fluid administration
    Alveolar ventilation
    Hypothermia

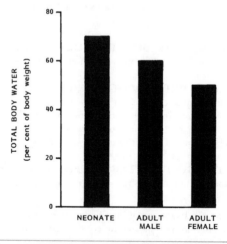

Fig. 21-1. *Total body water represents about 70% of the body weight (kg) of a neonate, 60% of an adult male, and 50% of an adult female. Anhydrous fat contributes a disproportionate amount to the body weight of an adult female, explaining the decreased amount of body water relative to body weight.*

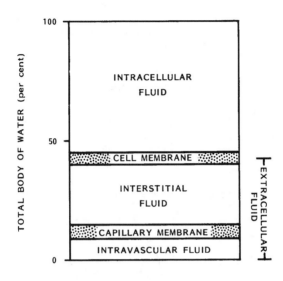

Fig. 21-2. *Total body water is designated as intracellular or extracellular fluid, depending on the location of water relative to the cell membrane. Water in the extracellular compartment is further subdivided as interstitial or intravascular (plasma) fluid, depending on its location relative to the capillary membrane. About 55% of total body water is intracellular, 37% is interstitial, and the remaining 8% is intravascular.*

Table 21-2. *Calculation of Total Body Water Content and Distribution in a 70-kg Adult*

	Male	Female
Total body water	42 L $(70 \times 0.6)^a$	35 L $(70 \times 0.5)^a$
Total intracellular water	23 L $(42 \times 0.55)^b$	19 L $(35 \times 0.55)^b$
Total extracellular water	19 L (42×0.45)	16 L (35×0.45)

[a] *Total body water content constitutes 60% of the body weight (kg) of an adult male and 50% of the body weight of an adult female.*
[b] *Intracellular water represents about 55% of the total body water content.*

Table 21-3. *Approximate Composition of Extracellular and Intracellular Fluid (mEq·L⁻¹)ᵃ*

	Extracellular		Intracellular
	Intravascular	Interstitial	
Sodium	140	145	10
Potassium	5	4	150
Calcium	5	2.5	<1
Magnesium	2	1.5	40
Chloride	103	115	4
Bicarbonate	28	30	10

ᵃ *Total anion concentration consists of phosphates, sulfates, organic acids, and negatively charged sites on proteins.*

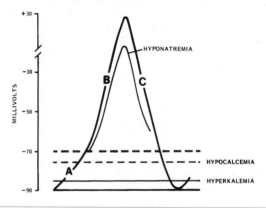

Fig. 21-3. *Schematic diagram of the action potential of an automatic (pacemaker) cell. The resting membrane potential (bottom solid line) is normally –90 mV. Continuous movement of sodium and potassium across the cell membrane results in spontaneous depolarization (A), until the threshold potential (thick dashed line) is reached at about –70 mV. When the threshold potential is reached, there is a sudden increase in permeability of the cell membrane to sodium. Rapid depolarization (B) leads to the production of an action potential. After propagation of the action potential, permeability of the cell membrane is restored, sodium is pumped out of the cell, and repolarization occurs (C). Disturbances of electrolyte concentrations alter the electrophysiology of the cell. For example, hyponatremia decreases the amplitude of the action potential. Hyperkalemia results in a less negative resting membrane potential. Hypocalcemia results in a more negative threshold potential.*

Table 21-4. *Signs and Symptoms of Hyponatremia Due to Increased Total Body Water Content*

Decreased hematocrit

Decreased serum osmolarity

Pulmonary edema

Confusion and drowsiness (serum sodium <120 mEq•L^{-1})

Seizures and coma (serum sodium <110 mEq•L^{-1})

Cardiac dysrhythmias (serum sodium <100 mEq•L^{-1})

results in water retention, low output of a highly concentrated urine, and dilutional hyponatremia (plasma osmolarity <280 mOsm•L^{-1}).

1. This syndrome has been described after a number of events, especially the postoperative period (ADH released for up to 96 hours postoperatively) (Table 21-5).

Table 21-5. *Factors Associated With Inappropriate Secretion of Antidiuretic Hormone*

Postoperative period

Positive pressure ventilation of the lungs

Endocrine disorders
    Adrenocortical insufficiency
    Anterior pituitary damage

Carcinoma of the lung

Central nervous system dysfunction
    Infection
    Hemorrhage
    Trauma

Drugs
    Chlorpropamide
    Opioids
    Diuretics
    Antimetabolites

  2. **Treatment** is a decrease in water intake to 500 ml·d^{-1}.
  D. **Management of anesthesia** is influenced by the likely presence of renal, cardiac, or liver disease as an etiology of excess body water and decreased excitability of cells due to the low plasma sodium concentration.

V. **TOTAL BODY WATER DEFICIT** results in **hypernatremia** (sodium concentration >145 mEq·L^{-1}), most often due to deficiencies or absence of ADH (diabetes insipidus) or resistance of renal tubules to the effects of this hormone.

  A. **Signs and symptoms** reflect loss of water from all fluid compartments, manifested as dehydration (dry mucous membranes, orthostatic hypotension).
  B. **Treatment** is administration of free water guided by changes in blood pressure, urine output, and measurement of the plasma sodium concentration (correct at a maximum rate of 0.5 mEq·L^{-1}·h^{-1}).
  C. **Management of anesthesia** is influenced by the likely presence of a decreased intravascular fluid volume due to a total body water deficit.

VI. **SODIUM EXCESS** (plasma sodium concentration >145 mEq·L^{-1})

  A. The kidneys closely regulate total body sodium content such that excess accumulation of sodium is almost impossible, unless there is impaired renal function (congestive heart failure, cirrhosis of the liver).
  B. **Signs and symptoms** are peripheral edema and hypertension due to the expanded intravascular fluid volume.
  C. **Treatment** is diuretic-induced facilitation of excretion of sodium by the kidneys.
  D. **Management of anesthesia** is not altered beyond the recognition that the intravascular fluid volume is likely to be increased.

VII. **SODIUM DEFICIT** (plasma sodium concentration <135 mEq·L^{-1})

  A. **Signs and symptoms** of total sodium deficit reflect the presence of a decreased intravascular fluid volume (low blood pressure, oliguria, increased hematocrit).
  B. **Treatment** is with hypertonic saline in symptomatic patients.

C. **Management of Anesthesia** (see section V C)

VIII. **HYPERKALEMIA** (plasma potassium concentration >5.5 mEq·L^{-1}) can be due to an **increased total body potassium content** or an **alteration in distribution of potassium** between intracellular and extracellular sites (Table 21-6).

A. **Signs and Symptoms**

  1. Adverse effects of hyperkalemia are more likely to accompany an acute increase in the plasma potassium concentration (cardiac conduction disturbances characterized by prolongation of the P-R interval, widening of the QRS complex, and peaking of the T wave on the electrocardiogram [ECG]) (Fig. 21-4).

  2. Chronic hyperkalemia is more likely to be associated with normalization of gradients across cell membranes and an absence of symptoms.

Table 21-6. *Causes of Hyperkalemia*

Increased Total Body Potassium Content
  Acute oliguric renal failure
  Chronic renal disease
  Hypoaldosteronism
  Drugs that impair potassium excretion
    Triamterene
    Spironolactone
    Nonsteroidal anti-inflammatory drugs
  Drugs that inhibit the renin-angiotensin-aldosterone system
    Beta antagonists
    Angiotensin-converting enzyme inhibitors

Altered Distribution of Potassium Between Intracellular and Extracellular Sites
  Succinylcholine
  Respiratory or metabolic acidosis
  Hemolysis
  Lysis of cells due to chemotherapy
  Iatrogenic bolus

Pseudohyperkalemia

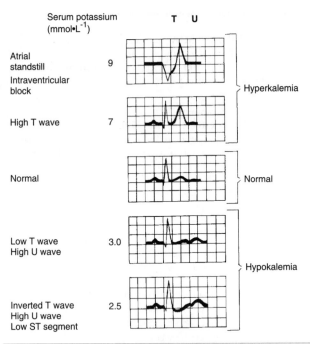

Fig. 21-4. *Manifestations on the electrocardiogram of changes in the plasma potassium concentration. (Goudsouzian NG, Karamanian A. The electrocardiogram. In: Physiology for the Anesthesiologist. E. Norwalk, CT. Appleton & Lange 1977;37, with permission.)*

    B. Treatment is indicated in the presence of ECG signs of hyperkalemia (Fig. 21-4) or in the presence of a plasma potassium concentration that is >6.5 mEq·L^{-1} (Table 21-7).

    C. Management of Anesthesia

        1. If it is not possible to lower the plasma potassium concentration to <5.5 mEq·L^{-1} before elective surgery, the anesthetic technique should be adjusted such that adverse effects of hyperkalemia are recognized intraoperatively (ECG) and the likelihood of any additional increase in the plasma potassium concentration is minimized (avoid hypoventilation).

        2. Succinylcholine-induced potassium release may be undesirable.

Table 21-7. *Treatment of Hyperkalemia*

	Dose	Mechanism	Onset	Duration
Calcium gluconate	10–20 ml of a 10% solution IV	Direct antagonism	Rapid	15–30 min
Sodium bicarbonate	50–100 mEq IV	Shift intracellular	15–30 min	3–6 h
Glucose and insulin	25–50 g with 10–20 units IV	Shift intracellular	15–30 min	3–6 h
Hyper-ventilation	$PaCO_2$ 25–30 mmHg	Shift intracellular	Rapid	
Kayexelate		Remove	1–3 h	
Peritoneal dialysis		Remove	1–3 h	
Hemodialysis		Remove	Rapid	

    3. The presence of potassium in crystalloid solutions for intravenous infusion is a consideration.

IX. PSEUDOHYPERKALEMIA is due to the in vitro (spurious) release of intracellular potassium.

X. HYPOKALEMIA (plasma potassium concentration <3.5 mEq·L^{-1}) can be due to a **decreased total body potassium content** or to **altered distribution of potassium** between intracellular and extracellular sites (Table 21-8). Stress-induced catecholamine release during the immediate preoperative period leading to beta-2-mediated translocation of potassium into intracellular sites may be responsible for acute decreases in the plasma potassium concentration.

    A. Signs and Symptoms (Table 21-9 and Fig. 21-4)

    B. Treatment depends on whether the decreased potassium concentration is associated with normal or decreased total body potassium content.

        1. Excessive hyperventilation of the lungs is corrected.

        2. Supplemental potassium chloride (0.2 mEq·kg^{-1}·h^{-1} IV) may be beneficial in severely depleted patients, recognizing that potassium content cannot be totally cor-

Table 21-8. *Causes of Hypokalemia*

Decreased Total Body Potassium Content
  Gastrointestinal loss
    Vomiting–diarrhea
    Nasogastric suction
    Villous adenoma of the colon
  Renal loss
    Osmotic or tubular diuretics
    Hyperglycemia
    Aldosteronism
    Excess endogenous or exogenous cortisol
    Surgical trauma
  Insufficient oral intake

Altered Distribution of Potassium Between Intracellular and Extracellular Sites
  Respiratory or metabolic alkalosis
  Glucose and insulin
  Familial periodic paralysis
  Beta-2 agonist stimulation
  Hypercalcemia
  Hypomagnesemia

Table 21-9. *Signs and Symptoms of Hypokalemia*

Skeletal muscle weakness (most prominent in legs)
Polyuria
Metabolic alkalosis
Orthostatic hypotension
Poor myocardial contractility (most likely to be associated with chronic hypokalemia)
Cardiac conduction disturbances (most likely to be associated with abrupt additional decreases in the plasma potassium concentration in the presence of chronic hypokalemia; increased automaticity terminating in ventricular fibrillation is common)

rected in the 12 to 24 hours preceding elective surgery.
C. Management of Anesthesia
  1. Advisability of proceeding with elective surgery in the

presence of chronic plasma potassium concentrations <3.5 mEq·L^{-1} is controversial.
2. Avoid glucose loads and hyperventilation of the lungs (guide by capnography and PaCO$_2$).
3. Responses to nondepolarizing muscle relaxants may be prolonged.
4. Choice of anesthetic drugs or techniques may be influenced by the association of chronic hypokalemia with decreased myocardial contractility, decreased sympathetic nervous system activity (orthostatic hypotension), and decreased urine concentrating ability (polyuria).
5. The ECG is monitored continuously for evidence of hypokalemia.

XI. **CALCIUM** is essential for nerve and skeletal muscle excitability (nonionized fraction is physiologically active and is bound by albumin).

A. **Hypercalcemia** (plasma calcium concentration >5.5 mEq·L^{-1}) is most often due to hyperparathyroidism or to neoplastic disease with bony metastases.
1. **Signs and Symptoms** (Table 21-10)
2. **Treatment** of hypercalcemia is diuresis (normal saline 150 ml·h^{-1} plus furosemide 1 to 2 mg·kg^{-1} IV) in the presence of central venons pressure monitoring.
3. **Management of Anesthesia.** The cardinal feature is maintenance of hydration and urine output with intravenous fluids containing sodium. Preoperative presence of skeletal muscle weakness suggests the possibility of decreased dose requirements for muscle relaxants.

Table 21-10. *Signs and Symptoms of Hypercalcemia*

Sedation
Vomiting
Polyuria
Cardiac conduction disturbances (prolonged P-R interval, wide QRS, shortened Q-T interval)
Renal calculi

B. **Hypocalcemia** (plasma calcium concentration <4.5 mEq·L^{-1}) is most often due to a decreased plasma albumin concentration, hypoparathyroidism, or renal failure.
   1. **Signs and Symptoms** (Table 21-11)
   2. **Treatment** is with the intravenous infusion of calcium and correction of any co-existing alkalosis.
   3. **Management of anesthesia.** Alkalosis due to hyperventilation of the lungs is avoided. Intraoperative hypotension may reflect exaggerated drug-induced cardiac depression in the presence of a decreased plasma ionized calcium concentration. Postoperatively, sudden decreases in the plasma calcium concentration can produce skeletal muscle spasm, including laryngospasm.

XII. **MAGNESIUM** is important in the regulation of presynaptic release of acetylcholine from nerve endings.

A. **Hypermagnesemia** (plasma magnesium concentration >2.5 mEq·L^{-1}) is most often due to renal failure or administration of magnesium to treat pregnancy-induced hypertension.
   1. **Signs and Symptoms** (Table 21-12)
   2. **Treatment** of acute manifestations of hypermagnesemia is the intravenous administration of calcium.
   3. **Management of anesthesia** includes avoidance of acidosis, maintenance of urine output, and recognition that responses to muscle relaxants may be prolonged.
B. **Hypomagnesemia** (plasma magnesium concentration <1.5 mEq·L^{-1}) is most often associated with chronic alcoholism, vomiting, and diarrhea.

Table 21-11. *Signs and Symptoms of Acute Hypocalcemia or Hypomagnesemia*

Numbness and circumoral paresthesias

Skeletal muscle spasm (laryngospasm)

Hypotension (decreased myocardial contractility)

Confusion

Seizures

Prolonged Q-T interval (not a consistent observation)

Table 21-12. *Signs and Symptoms of Hypermagnesemia*

> Central nervous system depression (hyporeflexia, sedation)
>
> Cardiac depression
>
> Skeletal muscle weakness (apnea)

1. **Signs and symptoms** (Table 21-11). Cardiac dysrhythmias attributed to diuretic-induced hypokalemia may be due to hypomagnesemia.
2. **Treatment** of hypomagnesemia is with intravenous administration of magnesium sulfate.

XIII. ACID-BASE DISTURBANCES are classified as respiratory or metabolic, based on the measurement of the arterial hydrogen ion concentration (pHa) and $PaCO_2$ and estimation of the plasma bicarbonate (HCO_3) concentration from a nomogram (Figs. 21-5 to 21-7).

   A. Respiratory acidosis is most often due to drug-induced depression of alveolar ventilation, disorders of neuromuscular function, and intrinsic lung disease (Fig. 21-6).

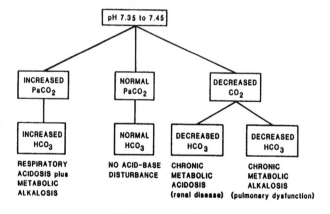

Fig. 21-5. *Diagnostic approach to the interpretation of a normal arterial pH based on the $PaCO_2$ and HCO_3 (bicarbonate) concentration.*

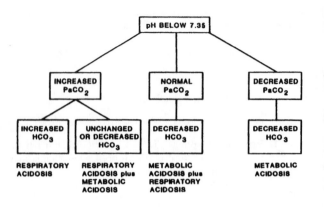

Fig. 21-6. *Diagnostic approach to the interpretation of an arterial pH <7.35 based on the $PaCO_2$ and HCO_3 (bicarbonate) concentration.*

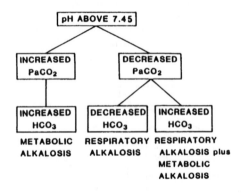

Fig. 21-7. *Diagnostic approach to the interpretation of an arterial pH >7.45 based on the $PaCO_2$ and HCO_3 (bicarbonate) concentration.*

1. **Treatment** of respiratory acidosis is by correction of the disorder responsible for hypoventilation.
2. Rapid lowering of a chronically elevated $PaCO_2$ will decrease body stores of carbon dioxide more rapidly

than the kidneys can excrete HCO_3, resulting in metabolic alkalosis (neuromuscular irritability, seizures).

B. Respiratory alkalosis is most often due to iatrogenic hyperventilation of the lungs during general anesthesia (Table 21-13).

    1. Treatment is directed at correction of the underlying disorder responsible for alveolar hyperventilation.

    2. Hypokalemia and hypochloremia that characterize respiratory alkalosis may also require treatment.

C. Metabolic acidosis is due to events that result in accumulation of nonvolatile acids (Table 21-14).

    1. Treatment of metabolic acidosis is with the intravenous administration of sodium bicarbonate.

    2. Sodium bicarbonate administration results in endogenous carbon dioxide production, necessitating an increase in alveolar ventilation to prevent hypercarbia and a worsening of the already existing acidosis.

Table 21-13. *Causes of Respiratory Alkalosis*

Iatrogenic

Decreased barometric pressure

Arterial hypoxemia

Central nervous system injury

Hepatic disease

Pregnancy

Salicylate overdose

Table 21-14. *Causes of Metabolic Acidosis*

Inadequate tissue oxygenation (lactic acidosis)

Renal failure

Diabetic ketoacidosis

Hepatic failure

Increased skeletal muscle activity

Cyanide poisoning

Carbon monoxide poisoning

Table 21-15. *Causes of Metabolic Alkalosis*

Vomiting

Nasogastric suction

Diuretic therapy

Iatrogenic

Hypovolemia

Hyperaldosteronism

Chloride-wasting diarrhea

D. Metabolic alkalosis is characterized by loss of nonvolatile acids from the extracellular fluid (Table 21-15).

1. Depletion of intravascular fluid volume is the most important factor in maintaining metabolic alkalosis.

2. Hypokalemia and skeletal muscle weakness are often present when hypovolemia complicates metabolic alkalosis.

CHAPTER 22

Endocrine Disease

An endocrine gland disorder (overproduction or underproduction of single or multiple hormones) may be the primary reason for surgery, or it may co-exist in a patient requiring an operation unrelated to endocrine gland dysfunction (see Stoelting RK, Dierdorf SF. Endocrine disease. In: Anesthesia and Co-Existing Disease. 3rd Ed. New York. Churchill Livingstone, 1993). The presence of unsuspected endocrine disease may be determined by seeking the answer to specific questions in the patient's preoperative evaluation (Table 22-1).

I. **DIABETES MELLITUS** is present as either insulin-dependent diabetes mellitus (IDDM) or non-insulin-dependent diabetes mellitus (NIDDM) in an estimated 2.4% of the U.S. population (Table 22-2).

  A. **Treatment** includes diet, oral hypoglycemic drugs, exogenous insulin, and, in select patients, transplantation of pancreatic tissue.

  1. **Oral Hypoglycemic Drugs** (Table 22-3)

    a. These drugs require the presence of functional pancreatic beta cells and thus are not effective in patients with IDDM.

    b. The most serious drug-induced complication is prolonged hypoglycemia, which is most likely to develop in a patient with renal disease.

  2. **Exogenous Insulin** (Table 22-4)

    a. Most diabetics require a combination of regular (rapid-acting) and Lente (intermediate-acting) insulin.

    b. Protamine-containing insulin preparations may place the patient at risk of the development of a life-threatening allergic reaction when protamine is administered to antagonize the anticoagulant effects of heparin.

    c. The use of tight metabolic control (blood glucose 75 to 125 mg·dl^{-1}) to prevent diabetic complications is controversial. The concentration of glycosylated hemoglobin is probably the best measure of overall blood glucose control.

Table 22-1. *Preoperative Evaluation of Endocrine Function*

Does urinalysis reveal glycosuria?

Are blood pressure and heart rate normal?

Is body weight unchanged?

Is sexual function normal?

Is there a history of medication with drugs relevant to endocrine function?

Table 22-2. *Classification of Diabetes Mellitus*

	IDDM	NIDDM
Age of onset (y)	<16	>35
Onset	Abrupt	Gradual
Manifestations	Polyphagia Polydipsia Polyuria	May be asymptomatic
Require exogenous insulin	Yes	Not always
Susceptibility to ketoacidosis	Yes	Not always
Blood glucose concentration	Wide fluctuations	Relatively stable
Nutrition	Thin	Obese
Microangiopathy	Common	Infrequent
Macroangiopathy	Infrequent	Common
Other autoimmune diseases present	Maybe	No

Table 22-3. *Oral Hypoglycemic Drugs*

Drug	Relative Potency	Duration of Action (h)
First generation		
Tolbutamine	1	6–10
Acetohexamide	2.5	12–18
Tolazamide	5	16–24
Chlorpropamide	6	24–72
Second generation		
Glyburide	150	18–24
Glipizide	100	16–24

Table 22-4. *Classification of Insulin Preparations*

	Hours After Subcutaneous Administration (Estimated)		
	Onset	Peak	Duration
Fast-acting			
Regular[a]	0.5–1	2–4	6–8
Semilente	1–3	5–10	16
Intermediate-acting			
Isophane (NPH)[a]	2–4	6–12	18–26
Lente[a]	2–4	6–12	18–26
Long-acting			
Protamine zinc	4–8	14–24	28–36
Ultralente	4–8	14–24	28–36

NPH, neutral (N) solution, protamine (P), with origin in Hagedorn's laboratory (H).
[a] Available as human insulin (Humulin).

B. Complications (Table 22-5)

C. Management of anesthesia for the diabetic patient undergoing elective surgery is intended to **mimic normal metabolism** by (1) avoiding hypoglycemia (provide exogenous glucose); and (2) preventing excessive hyperglycemia, ketoacidosis, and electrolyte disturbances (provide exogenous insulin).

1. **Preoperative Evaluation**

   a. The well-controlled diet-treated patient with NIDDM does not require prior hospitalization or any special treatment (including insulin) either before or during surgery. Likewise, the patient with well-controlled IDDM undergoing a brief outpatient surgical procedure may not require any adjustment in the usual subcutaneous insulin regimen. If an oral hypoglycemic drug is being administered, it may be continued until the evening before surgery.

   b. Preadmission to the hospital is probably indicated only for the patient with poorly controlled IDDM.

   c. Known complications of diabetes are considered in the preoperative preparation (Table 22-5).

2. **Exogenous Insulin.** There is a consensus that the patient with IDDM who is undergoing major surgery

Table 22-5. *Complications of Diabetes Mellitus*

Ketoacidosis

Atherosclerosis
  Cerebrovascular accident
  Myocardial infarction
  Cardiomyopathy

Microangiopathy
  Retinopathy (laser photocoagulation)
  Nephropathy (renal transplantation)

Autonomic neuropathy
  Orthostatic hypotension
  Resting tachycardia
  Gastroparesis (vomiting, diarrhea)
  Impotence
  Cardiac dysrhythmias
  Asymptomatic hypoglycemia
  Sudden death syndrome (may occur coincident-
    ally during the perioperative period)

Sensory neuropathy
  Nocturnal discomfort in extremities
  Carpal tunnel syndrome

Stiff joint syndrome (difficult exposure of the glottic
  opening)

Scleredema

should be treated with insulin, but the accepted route of administration (subcutaneous, intravenous) remains unsettled.

a. The **traditional** approach is subcutaneous administration of one-fourth to one-half the usual daily intermediate-acting dose of insulin on the morning of surgery. If regular insulin is part of the morning schedule, the intermediate-acting insulin dose may be increased 0.5 unit for each unit of regular insulin. An intravenous infusion of glucose (5 to 10 $g \cdot h^{-1}$) is initiated at the same time to minimize the likelihood of hypoglycemia.

b. **Continuous intravenous infusion** of insulin is an alternative to the traditional approach, especially in diabetic patients undergoing prolonged and stressful surgery, such as cardiopulmonary bypass (Table 22-6).

Table 22-6. *Continuous Intravenous Infusion of Regular Insulin During the Perioperative Period*

1. Mix 50 units of regular insulin in 500 ml normal saline (1 unit•h^{-1} = 10 ml•h^{-1})
2. Initiate intravenous infusion at 0.5–1 unit•h^{-1}
3. Measure blood glucose concentration as necessary (usually every hour), and adjust insulin infusion rate accordingly:

<80 mg•dl^{-1}	Turn infusion off for 30 minutes Administer 25 ml of 50% glucose Remeasure blood glucose concentration in 30 minutes
80–120 mg•dl^{-1}	Decrease insulin infusion by 0.3 unit•h^{-1}
120–180 mg•dl^{-1}	No change in insulin infusion rate
180– 220 mg•dl^{-1}	Increase insulin infusion by 0.3 unit•h^{-1}
>220 mg•dl^{-1}	Increase insulin infusion by 0.5 unit•h^{-1}

4. Provide sufficient glucose (5–10 g•h^{-1}) and potassium (2–4 mEq•h^{-1})

(Data from Hirsch IB, Magill JB, Cryer PE, White PF. Perioperative management of surgical patients with diabetes mellitus. Anesthesiology 1991;74:346–59.)

    c. Monitoring blood glucose every hour during the time in the operating room is often recommended. Values <100 mg•dl^{-1} and >250 mg•dl^{-1} are typically treated with additional glucose or exogenous insulin, respectively.

   3. Induction and Maintenance. Choice of drugs for induction and maintenance of anesthesia is less important than monitoring the blood glucose concentration (see section I C2c) and treatment of potential physiologic derangements associated with diabetes (Table 22-5).

  D. Emergency Surgery. It is useful to evaluate the patient's metabolic status (blood glucose concentration, electrolytes, pH, urine ketones) before proceeding with anesthesia.

  E. Hyperosmolar Hyperglycemic Nonketotic Coma (Table 22-7)

II. INSULINOMA. The principal challenge during anesthesia for surgical excision of an insulinoma is maintenance of

Table 22-7. *Hyperosmolar Hyperglycemic Nonketotic Coma*

Hyperosmolarity (>330 mOsm•L^{-1})
Hyperglycemia (>600 mg•dl^{-1})
Normal pH
Osmotic diuresis (hypokalemia)
Hypovolemia (hemoconcentration)
Central nervous system dysfunction

a normal blood glucose concentration (profound hypoglycemia during manipulation of the tumor and hyperglycemia after its removal).

III. THYROID GLAND DYSFUNCTION

A. **Thyroid function tests** are used to assess the rate of production of triiodothyronine (T_3) and/or thyroxine (T_4) in the detection of hyperthyroidism and hypothyroidism (Tables 22-8 and 22-9).

Table 22-8. *Tests of Thyroid Gland Function*

Test	Purpose
Total plasma thyroxine (T_4) level	Detects >90% of hyperthyroid patients; influenced by level of T_4-binding globulin (see Table 22-9)
Resin triiodothyronine uptake (RT$_3$U)	Clarifies whether changes in T_4 level are due to thyroid gland dysfunction or alterations in T_4-binding globulin
Total plasma triiodothyronine (T_3) level	Confirms diagnosis of hyperthyroidism; may be low in absence of hypothyroidism in patients who are cirrhotic, uremic, or malnourished
Thyroid stimulating hormone (TSH) level	Confirms diagnosis of primary hypothyroidism; may be increased before T_4 level is decreased

(Continues)

Table 22-8. *Tests of Thyroid Gland Function* (Continued)

Test	Purpose
Thyroid scan	Demonstrates iodide-concentrating capacity of thyroid gland; functioning thyroid gland tissue rarely malignant
Ultrasonography	Discriminates between cystic (rarely malignant) and solid (may be malignant) nodules
Antibodies to thyroid gland components	Distinguishes Hashimoto's thyroiditis from cancer

Table 22-9. *Differential Diagnosis of Thyroid Gland Dysfunction*[a]

Condition	T$_4$	RT$_3$U	T$_3$	TSH
Hyperthyroidism	Increased	Increased	Increased	Normal
Primary hypothyroidism	Decreased	Decreased	Decreased	Increased
Secondary hypothyroidism	Decreased	Decreased	Decreased	Decreased
Pregnancy	Increaed	Decreased	Normal	Normal

[a] See Table 22-8 for definitions.

B. **Hyperthyroidism**
  1. **Signs and Symptoms** (Table 22-10)
  2. **Treatment** mandates that the patient be followed indefinitely for the onset of hypothyroidism or recurrence of hyperthyroidism (Table 22-11).
  3. **Thyroid storm** (thyrotoxicosis) is an abrupt exacerbation of hyperthyroidism (may occur during the operative or early postoperative period), manifested as hyperthermia, tachycardia, congestive heart failure, dehydration, and shock. Treatment is infusion of cooled saline solutions and continuous infusion of esmolol to maintain the heart rate at an acceptable level. When hypotension is persistent, the administration of cortisol (100 to 200 mg IV) may be considered.
  4. **Management of Anesthesia** (Table 22-12)

Table 22-10. *Signs and Symptoms of Hyperthyroidism*

Sign/Symptom	Incidence (% of patients)
Goiter	100
Tachycardia	100
Anxiety	99
Tremor	97
Heat intolerance	89
Fatigue	88
Weight loss	85
Eye signs	71
Skeletal muscle weakness	70
Atrial fibrillation	10

Table 22-11. *Treatment of Hyperthyroidism*

Antithyroid Drugs
Propylthiouracil
Methimazole
Propranolol (alleviates symptoms of excessive sympathetic nervous system activity)

Subtotal Thyroidectomy
Prepare for surgery with a beta antagonist
Damage to recurrent laryngeal nerve may occur (hoarseness, aspiration)
Airway obstruction (tracheomalacia, hematoma)
Hypoparathyroidism (laryngospasm may be first evidence of hypocalcemia)

Radioactive Iodine
Avoids risk of anesthesia and surgery
Treatment of choice in patient >40 years of age

C. **Hypothyroidism** is estimated to be present in 0.5% to 0.8% of the population. Subclinical hypothyroidism manifesting only as an increased thyroid stimulating hormone (TSH) concentration is present in 5% of the population, with a prevalence of 13.2% in otherwise healthy elderly patients, especially females.

Table 22-12. *Management of Anesthesia in the Patient With Hyperthyroidism*

Render euthyroid before elective surgery (when cannot delay, control hyperdynamic cardiovascular system with esmolol)

Avoid anticholinergic drug in preoperative medication

Evaluate upper airway for obstruction from goiter (computed tomography)

Induction of anesthesia (thiopental plus succinylcholine or nondepolarizing drug that lacks cardiovascular effects)

Maintenance of anesthesia (isoflurane–nitrous oxide; anesthetic requirements not greatly altered)

Monitor for signs of thyroid storm (temperature, heart rate)

Treatment of hypotension (possible exaggerated response to indirect acting vasopressor)

Regional anesthesia a consideration as blocks portion of the sympathetic nervous system

1. **Signs and Symptoms.** The onset of hypothyroidism in the adult patient is insidious and may go unrecognized (Table 22-13). Cardiovascular impairment is minimal to absent in the presence of subclinical hypothyroidism.
2. **Treatment** is with oral administration of thyroxine. It is not unusual to encounter patients who have been previously started on thyroid hormone replacement with-

Table 22-13. *Signs and Symptoms of Hypothyroidism*

Lethargy

Intolerance to cold

Bradycardia

Peripheral vasoconstriction (conserve heat)

Atrophy of the adrenal cortex

Hyponatremia

out firm laboratory confirmation of hypothyroidism.

3. **Management of anesthesia** should consider possible adverse responses associated with hypothyroidism (Table 22-14).

   a. Controlled clinical studies do not confirm an increased risk to patients with mild to moderate hypothyroidism who are undergoing elective surgery.

   b. **Preoperative Medication.** Supplemental cortisol may be considered.

   c. **Induction of anesthesia** is often with intravenous administration of ketamine.

   d. **Maintenance of anesthesia** is often achieved by inhalation of nitrous oxide plus supplementation, if necessary, with a short-acting opioid, benzodiazepine, or ketamine. At the conclusion of surgery, removal of the tracheal tube is deferred until the patient is responding appropriately and body temperature is near 37°C.

Table 22-14. *Possible Adverse Responses of the Hypothyroid Patient During the Perioperative Period*

Increased sensitivity to depressant drugs

Hypodynamic cardiovascular system
   Decreased heart rate
   Decreased cardiac output

Slowed metabolism of drugs

Unresponsive baroreceptor reflexes

Impaired ventilatory responses to arterial hypoxemia or hypercarbia

Hypovolemia

Delayed gastric emptying time

Hyponatremia

Hypothermia

Anemia

Hypoglycemia

Adrenal insufficiency

     e. Regional anesthesia is an appropriate selection, provided intravascular fluid volume is well maintained.

IV. PARATHYROID GLAND DYSFUNCTION

  A. Primary hyperparathyroidism results from excessive secretion of parathyroid hormone due to a benign parathyroid adenoma (responsible for 90% of affected patients), carcinoma of a parathyroid gland, or hyperplasia of the parathyroid glands.

    1. Signs and Symptoms (Table 22-15)

    2. Treatment of hypercalcemia is diuresis (normal saline 150 ml·h^{-1} plus furosemide 1 to 2 mg·kg^{-1} IV) in the presence of central venous pressure monitoring.

      a. A thiazide diuretic is not recommended, as these

Table 22-15. *Signs and Symptoms of Hypercalcemia Due to Hyperparathyroidism*

System	Signs/Symptoms
Neuromuscular	Skeletal muscle weakness
Renal	Renal stones Polyuria and polydipsia Decreased glomerular filtration rate
Hematopoietic	Anemia
Cardiac	Hypertension Prolonged P-R interval Short Q-T interval
Gastrointestinal	Abdominal pain Vomiting Peptic ulcer Pancreatitis
Skeletal	Skeletal demineralization Pathologic fractures Collapse of vertebral bodies
Nervous system	Somnolence Psychosis Decreased pain sensation
Ocular	Calcifications (band keratopathy) Conjunctivitis

drugs may unpredictably increase the plasma calcium concentration.

    b. Definitive treatment of primary hyperparathyroidism is surgical removal of the diseased or abnormal portions of the parathyroid glands.

  3. Management of Anesthesia. There is no evidence that a specific anesthetic drug or technique is indicated.

    a. Maintenance of hydration and urine output is important in the perioperative management of hypercalcemia.

    b. Somnolence and skeletal muscle weakness suggest a possible decreased requirement for anesthetic drugs and muscle relaxants.

B. Hypoparathyroidism is most often due to accidental removal of the parathyroid glands, as during thyroidectomy. A plasma calcium concentration <4.5 m Eq·L^{-1} is the most valuable diagnostic indicator of hypoparathyroidism.

  1. Signs and symptoms depend on rapidity of onset of hypocalcemia. (Table 22-16).

  2. Treatment of acute hypocalcemia is with 10 ml of 10% calcium gluconate IV until signs of neuromuscular irritability disappear.

  3. Management of Anesthesia (see Chapter 21, XI B3)

C. DiGeorge Syndrome (congenital thymic hypoplasia) is characterized by hypoplasia of the parathyroid gland and thymic gland, resulting in hypocalcemia and the propensity to develop infections. Associated anomalies may include congenital heart disease and micrognathia.

Table 22-16. *Signs and Symptoms of Hypocalcemia Due to Hypoparathyroidism*

Acute Hypocalcemia (surgical removal)
  Perioral paresthesias
  Restlessness
  Neuromuscular irritability (positive Chvostek or
    Trousseau sign, inspiratory stridor)

Chronic Hypocalcemia (renal failure)
  Fatigue
  Skeletal muscle weakness
  Prolonged Q-T interval
  Cataracts

V. ADRENAL GLAND DYSFUNCTION

A. **Hyperadrenocorticism** (Cushing's disease)
   1. **Signs and Symptoms** (Table 22-17)
   2. **Treatment.** Transsphenoidal microadenomectomy is the preferred treatment for hyperadrenocorticism owing to excess secretion of adrenocorticotrophic hormone (ACTH) by the anterior pituitary.
   3. **Management of anesthesia** is influenced by the physiologic effects of excess cortisol secretion, especially as reflected on blood pressure, electrolyte balance, and blood glucose concentration. Osteoporosis is a consideration in positioning for the operative procedure. The plasma cortisol concentration decreases promptly after microadenomectomy or bilateral adrenalectomy. Initiation of intraoperative replacement therapy (cortisol 100 mg·d^{-1} IV) is recommended.

B. **Hypoadrenocorticism**
   1. **Signs and Symptoms** (Table 22-18)
   2. **Treatment** of life-threatening hypoadrenocorticism is administration of cortisol 100 mg IV, followed by continuous intravenous infusion of 10 mg·h^{-1}.
   3. **Surgery and Suppression of the Pituitary Adrenal Axis.** Corticosteroid supplementation should be increased in any patient being treated for chronic hypoadrenocorticism who is undergoing a surgical procedure. More controversial is the management of the patient who

---

Table 22-17. *Signs and Symptoms of Hyperadrenocorticism*

Hypertension
Hypokalemia
Hyperglycemia
Skeletal muscle weakness
Osteoporosis
Obesity
Hirsutism
Menstrual disturbances
Poor wound healing
Susceptibility to infection

Table 22-18. *Signs and Symptoms of Hypoadrenocorticism*

Weight loss

Skeletal muscle weakness

Hypotension (indistinguishable from shock due to loss of intravascular fluid volume)

Hyperkalemia

Hypoglycemia

Hyperpigmentation over palmar surfaces and pressure points

manifests suppression of the pituitary adrenal axis, owing to current or previous administration of a corticosteroid (dose or duration of therapy to produce suppression or the time necessary for recovery is not known) for a disease (asthma, rheumatoid arthritis) unrelated to pathology in the anterior pituitary or adrenal cortex.

   a. A clinical approach is often to administer empirically a supplemental dose of a corticosteroid (cortisol 25 mg IV at induction and 100 mg IV over the next 24 hours), when surgery is planned in a patient being treated with a corticosteroid or who has been treated for >1 month during the immediately preceding 6 to 12 months.

   b. A cause-effect relationship between intraoperative hypotension and acute hypoadrenocorticism in a patient previously treated with a corticosteroid has never been documented.

C. Hyperaldosteronism is suggested by diastolic hypertension in the presence of hypokalemic metabolic alkalosis and associated skeletal muscle weakness.

   1. Treatment is initially with supplemental potassium and administration of a competitive aldosterone antagonist such as spironolactone. Definitive treatment for an aldosterone-secreting tumor is surgical excision.

   2. Management of anesthesia is facilitated by preoperative correction of hypokalemia and treatment of hypertension. Orthostatic hypotension detected during the preoperative evaluation is a clue to unexpected hypovolemia in these patients. Supplementation with exogenous cortisol is a consideration.

D. Hypoaldosteronism is suggested by the presence of hyperkalemia in the absence of renal insufficiency.

E. Pheochromocytoma is a catecholamine-secreting tumor that may occur independently or as part of an autosomal dominant multiglandular neoplastic syndrome (Table 22-19).

1. **Diagnosis** of pheochromocytoma requires chemical confirmation of excessive catecholamine secretion (Table 22-20). Computed tomography is the initial localizing procedure in the diagnosis of pheochromocytoma.

2. **Signs and Symptoms.** The hallmark of pheochromocytoma is paroxysmal hypertension. The **triad of diaphoresis, tachycardia, and headache** in a hypertensive patient is highly suggestive of pheochromocytoma. Death resulting from a pheochromocytoma is often due to congestive heart failure, myocardial infarction, or intracerebral hemorrhage.

3. **Treatment** is surgical excision of the catecholamine secreting tumor only after medical control is optimized by institution of alpha blockade (phentolamine, prazosin, labetalol) and possibly beta blockade.

4. **Management of anesthesia** for the patient requiring excision of a pheochromocytoma is based on adminis-

Table 22-19. *Manifestations of Multiple Endocrine Neoplasia (MEN)*

Syndrome	Manifestations
MEN type IIa (Sipple syndrome)	Medullary thyroid cancer Parathyroid adenoma Pheochromocytoma
MEN type IIb	Medullary thyroid cancer Mucosal adenomas Marfan appearance Pheochromocytoma
von Hippel-Lindau syndrome	Hemangioblastoma involving the central nervous system Pheochromocytoma

Table 22-20. *Urinary Excretion of Catecholamines and Catecholamine Metabolites*

	Daily Urinary Excretion	
	Normal	Pheochromocytoma
Total metanephrines	0.1–1.6 mg	2.5–4 mg
Vanillylmandelic acid	1.8 mg	10–250 mg
Norepinephrine	<100 µg	
Epinephrine	<1 µg	
Total catecholamines	4–126 µg	200–4000 µg

tration of drugs that do not stimulate the sympathetic nervous system plus the use of invasive monitoring techniques (Table 22-21). Regional anesthesia is not protective, as postsynaptic alpha receptors can still respond to sudden increases in the circulating concentration of catecholamines.

VI. DYSFUNCTION OF THE TESTES OR OVARIES
(Table 22-22)

VII. PITUITARY GLAND DYSFUNCTION

A. **Acromegaly** is due to excess secretion of growth hormone in an adult, most often from an adenoma in the anterior pituitary gland.
   1. **Signs and Symptoms** (Table 22-23)
   2. **Management of anesthesia** must consider the potential for difficult upper airway management and anticipation of the possible need to insert a small-diameter tracheal tube. In placing a catheter in the radial artery, it is important to consider the possibility of inadequate collateral circulation at the wrist. Monitoring of the plasma glucose concentration is useful if diabetes mellitus accompanies acromegaly.

B. **Diabetes insipidus** reflects the absence of antidiuretic hormone, owing to the destruction of the posterior pituitary (neurogenic diabetes insipidus) or failure of the renal tubules to respond to the hormone (nephrogenic diabetes insipidus). **Treatment** is intravenous infusion of elec-

Table 22-21. *Management of Anesthesia for Excision of a Pheochromocytoma*

Continue alpha and beta antagonist therapy

Consider need for supplemental cortisol

Place intra-arterial catheter

Intravenous induction of anesthesia, followed by establishment of surgical level of anesthesia with isoflurane (desflurane or sevoflurane may be alternatives)

Skeletal muscle paralysis with a nondepolarizing muscle relaxant devoid of circulatory effects

Minimize circulatory responses to direct laryngoscopy and tracheal intubation (see Table 5-7)

Maintenance of anesthesia with isoflurane and nitrous oxide plus nitroprusside, esmolol, lidocaine, and phenylephrine as needed

Pulmonary artery catheter often recommended

Monitor arterial blood gases, electrolytes, blood glucose concentration

Postoperatively continue invasive monitoring and provide pain relief (neuraxial opioids)

Table 22-22. *Dysfunction of the Testes or Ovaries*

Klinefelter syndrome (XXY chromosomal defect, most common expression of testicular dysfunction)

Physiologic menopause (absence of estrogen leads to osteoporosis)

Premenstrual syndrome (prostaglandins)

Oral contraception (platelet aggregation increased by all these drugs)

Ovarian hyperstimulation syndrome (ascites, hypovolemia)

Turner syndrome (primary amenorrhea, difficult airway management)

Noonan syndrome (resembles Turner syndrome but mental retardation and congenital heart disease likely)

Stein-Leventhal syndrome (primary amenorrhea, hirsutism, and increased skeletal muscle development)

Table 22-23. *Manifestations of Acromegaly*

Paraseallar
Enlarged sella turcica
Headache
Visual field defects
Rhinorrhea

Excess Growth Hormone
Skeletal overgrowth (prognathism)
Soft tissue overgrowth (lips, tongue, epiglottis,
vocal cords)
Connective tissue overgrowth (recurrent laryngeal
nerve paralysis)
Peripheral neuropathy (carpal tunnel syndrome)
Visceromegaly
Glucose intolerance
Osteoarthritis
Osteoporosis
Hyperhydrosis
Skeletal muscle weakness

trolyte solutions if oral intake cannot offset polyuria. Chlorpropamide is useful in the treatment of nephrogenic diabetes insipidus, whereas intramuscular or intranasal vasopressin is useful for the management of neurogenic diabetes insipidus.

C. **Inappropriate secretion of antidiuretic hormone** accompanies diverse pathologic processes (intracranial tumors, hypothyroidism, carcinoma of the lung) and is common after surgery. An inappropriately increased urinary sodium concentration and osmolarity in the presence of hyponatremia and decreased plasma osmolarity is diagnostic. Initial treatment is restriction of fluid intake.

CHAPTER 23

Metabolic and Nutritional Disorders

An absence of a specific enzyme is often the reason for the occurrence of a metabolic disorder, whereas excess caloric intake is the likely cause of the common nutritional disorder, obesity (Table 23-1) (see Stoelting RK, Dierdorf SF. Metabolic and nutritional disorders. In: Anesthesia and Co-Existing Disease. 3rd Ed. New York. Churchill Livingstone, 1993).

I. **PORPHYRIAS** are a group of inborn errors of metabolism characterized by the overproduction of porphyria compounds and their precursors (Table 23-2).

   A. **Acute intermittent porphyria** reflects the accumulation of excessive amounts of porphobilinogen.

      1. **Signs and symptoms** include severe abdominal pain and neurotoxicity (psychoses, cranial nerves, autonomic nervous system, peripheral nervous system).

      2. **Prevention and Treatment** (Table 23-3)

      3. **Management of anesthesia** is designed to avoid administration of drugs that might provoke an acute attack (Table 23-4).

         a. Selection of regional anesthesia may be influenced by the presence of co-existing peripheral neuropathies.

         b. Perioperative monitoring should consider the frequent presence of autonomic nervous system dysfunction and the possibility of labile blood pressure.

         c. Weakened muscles of respiration and impaired swallowing owing to cranial nerve involvement may necessitate prolonged tracheal intubation and mechanical support of ventilation.

   B. **Porphyria cutanea tarda** is characterized by photosensitivity (avoid ultraviolet light and tape and pressure from a face mask) and the likely presence of co-existing liver disease. Anesthesia is not a hazard, and neurotoxicity is not present.

II. **GOUT** is a disorder of purine metabolism characterized by hyperuricemia and recurrent acute arthritis.

Table 23-1. *Metabolic and Nutritional Disorders*

Metabolic
Porphyria
Gout
Pseudogout
Hyperlipidemia
Carbohydrate metabolism disorders
Amino acid metabolism disorders
Mucopolysaccharidoses
Gangliosidoses

Nutritional
Morbid obesity
Obesity hypoventilation syndrome
Malnutrition
Anorexia nervosa
Vitamin imbalance disorders

Table 23-2. *Classification of Porphyria*

Hepatic Porphyrias
Acute intermittent porphyria
Porphyria cutanea tarda
Variegate porphyria
Hereditary coproporphyria

Erythropoietic Porphyrias
Erythropoietic uroporphyria
Erythropoietic protoporphyria

Table 23-3. *Prevention and Treatment of Acute Intermittent Porphyria*

Prevention (avoid starvation, dehydration, sepsis, and triggering drugs)

Treatment (prompt administration of hematin and glucose)
Opioids
Beta antagonist
Mechanical ventilation of the lungs
Nasogastric suction

Table 23-4. *Safe and Unsafe Drugs for Administration to a Patient With Acute Intermittent Porphyria*

Safe Drugs	Unsafe Drugs
Anticholinergics	Barbiturates
Anticholinesterases	Ethyl alcohol
Depolarizing and nondepolarizing muscle relaxants	Etomidate
	Phenytoin
Droperidol	Pentazocine
Opioids	Corticosteroids
Nitrous oxide	Imipramine
Volatile anesthetics	Tolbutamide
Propofol	Benzodiazepines(?)
Benzodiazepines(?)	Ketamine(?)
Ketamine(?)	

A. **Management of Anesthesia** (Table 23-5)
B. Despite appropriate precautions, acute attacks of gout often follow surgical procedures.

III. **LESCH-NYHAN SYNDROME** is a genetically determined disorder of purine metabolism manifesting exclusively in males as mental retardation, spasticity, and self-mutilation (oral scarring).

Table 23-5. *Management of Anesthesia in the Presence of Gout*

Prehydration

Evaluate renal function

Consider co-existing diseases
    Hypertension
    Ischemic heart disease
    Diabetes mellitus

Possibility of temporomandibular arthritis

Adverse effects of drug therapy

IV. HYPERLIPOPROTEINEMIA (Table 23-6)

V. CARNITINE DEFICIENCY may manifest as recurrent attacks of nausea and vomiting (systemic form) or skeletal muscle weakness and cardiomyopathy (myopathic form). Intravenous infusion of glucose is included in the perioperative management of these patients.

VI. DISORDERS OF CARBOHYDRATE METABOLISM (Table 23-7)

VII. DISORDERS OF AMINO ACID METABOLISM (Table 23-8)

Table 23-6. *Characteristics of Hyperlipoproteinemias*

	Cholesterol	Triglyceride	Xanthomas	Risk of Ischemic Heart Disease
Familial lipo-protein lipase deficiency (hyperchylo-micronemia)	Normal	Increased	Eruptive	Very low
Familial dys-betalipopro-teinemia	Increased	Increased	Palmar Planar Tendon	Very high
Familial hyper-cholesterole-mia	Increased	Normal to increased	Tendon	Very high
Familial hyper-triglyceride-mia	Normal	Increased	Eruptive	Low
Familial combined hyperlipide-mia	Markedly increased	Markedly increased	Palmar Planar Tendon	High
Polygenic hyperchole-sterolemia	Increased	Normal	Tendon	Moderate

Table 23-7. *Disorders of Carbohydrate Metabolism*

> von Gierke's disease (cannot convert glycogen to glucose and hypoglycemia may be profound)
>
> Pompe's disease (glycogen deposition in heart and upper airway)
>
> McArdle's disease (myoglobinuria may lead to renal failure)
>
> Galactosemia (cataracts, cirrhosis of liver, and mental retardation reflect tissue accumulation of galactose)
>
> Fructose 1,6-diphosphate deficiency (hypoglycemia, metabolic acidosis, and skeletal muscle hypotonia are common; use of lactated Ringer's solution is questionable)
>
> Pyruvate dehydrogenase deficiency (chronic metabolic acidosis; use of lactated Ringer's solution questionable)

VIII. MUCOPOLYSACCHARIDOSES (Table 23-9)

IX. GANGLIOSIDOSES are characterized by progressive neurodegeneration. Gaucher's disease is due to an inherited deficiency of the enzyme necessary to degrade glycolipids, leading to the accumulation of glucocerebroside in tissues.

X. MORBID OBESITY as reflected by weight >20% above the ideal weight is present in about 25% of the population.

    A. Treatment of obesity includes decreased caloric intake combined with exercise, very-low-calorie liquid protein diets (requires medical supervision) and consideration of gastroplasty.

    B. Adverse Effects (Table 23-10)

    C. Management of Anesthesia (Table 23-11)

XI. OBESITY HYPOVENTILATION SYNDROME (pickwickian syndrome) is characterized by massive obesity, daytime somnolence, and hypoventilation (eventually leads to pulmonary hypertension and right ventricular failure).

Table 23-8. Disorders of Amino Acid Metabolism

Disorder	Retardation	Seizures	Metabolic Acidosis	Hyper-ammon-emia	Hepatic Failure	Thrombo-embolism	Other
Phenylketonuria	Yes	Yes	No	No	No	No	
Homocystinuria	Yes/No	Yes	No	No	No	Yes	
Hypervalinemia	Yes	Yes	Yes	No	No	No	Hypoglycemia
Citrullinemia	Yes	Yes	No	Yes	Yes	No	
Branched chain aciduria (maple syrup urine disease)	Yes	Yes	Yes	No	Yes	Yes	
Methylmalonyl-coenzyme A mutase deficiency			Yes	Yes			Avoid nitrous oxide?
Isoleucinemia	Yes	Yes	Yes	Yes	Yes	No	
Methioninemia	Yes	No	No	No	No	No	Thermal instability
Histidinuria	Yes	Yes/No	No	No	No	No	Erythrocyte fragility
Neutral aminoaciduria (Hartnup disease)	Yes/No	Yes	Yes	No	No	No	Dermatitis
Arginemia	Yes		No	Yes	Yes	No	

Table 23-9. *Mucopolysaccharidoses*

Type	Eponym	Incidence	Clinical Features
I (H)	Hurler	1/100,000	Progressive involvement of heart, skeleton, and airways Progressive mental retardation Possible cervical spine involvement
I (S) (former-ly V)	Scheie	1/500,000	Cardiac valve involvement likely Slowly progressive skeletal and airway involvement Intellect usually normal
I (HG)	Hurler/Scheie	1/115,000	Mental retardation Micrognathia common
II	Hunter	1/110,000	Mild to severe forms Slowly progressive
III (A to D)	Sanfi-lippo	1/24,000 (?)	Progressive mental retardation Several enzyme deficiencies
IV (A, B)	Morquio	Rare	Intellect usually normal Odontoid hypoplasia common Pectus carinatum common Aortic valve disease common
VI	Maro-teaux–Lamy	Rare	Intellect usually normal Possible odontoid hypoplasia

Table 23-10. *Adverse Effects of Obesity*

Systemic hypertension
Hypercholesterolemia
Hypertriglyceridemia
Diabetes mellitus
Ischemic heart disease
Cardiomegaly
Pulmonary hypertension
Congestive heart failure
Restrictive ventilation defect
Arterial hypoxemia
Sleep apnea
Fatty liver infiltration
Osteoarthritis

Table 23-11. *Management of Anesthesia in the Presence of Obesity*

Preoperative Evaluation (Table 23-10)

Induction of Anesthesia
  Increased risk of pulmonary aspiration
  Decreased mandibular and cervical spine mobility
    (consider awake fiberoptic tracheal intubation
  Consider pharmacologic manipulation of gastric
    fluid pH and volume
  Maximize oxygen content of lungs before produc-
    ing apnea

Maintenance of Anesthesia
  Volatile anesthetic metabolism may be increased
    (fatty liver infiltration)
  Regional anesthesia may be technically difficult

Management of Ventilation
  Large tidal volume
  Prone and head-down position may further
    decrease PaO_2

Postoperative Complications
  Wound infection
  Deep vein thrombosis
  Pulmonary complications (semisitting position rec-
    ommended)

XII. **BULIMIA NERVOSA** is characterized by episodes of binge eating that occurs most often in females. Drug abuse is frequent in this patient group.

XIII. **ANOREXIA NERVOSA** is accompanied by autonomic nervous system changes (orthostatic hypotension, cardiac dysrhythmias), decreased myocardial contractility, thrombocytopenia, and anemia.

  A. **Treatment** may include enteral nutrition.
  B. **Management of anesthesia** includes consideration of electrolyte abnormalities, hypovolemia, cardiac dysfunction, and delayed gastric emptying time.

XIV. **MALNUTRITION** is responsive to caloric support as provided by enteral (when gastrointestinal tract is functioning) or total parenteral nutrition (Table 23-12).

Table 23-12. *Complications Associated With Total Parenteral Nutrition*

Hyperglycemia

Nonketotic hyperosmolar hyperglycemic coma

Hypoglycemia

Hyperchloremic metabolic acidosis

Fluid overload

Increased carbon dioxide production

Catheter-related sepsis

Electrolyte abnormalities

Renal dysfunction

Hepatic dysfunction

Thrombosis of central veins

Table 23-13. *Disorders Related to Vitamin Imbalance*

Thiamine deficiency (high-output congestive heart failure with mental confusion and polyneuropathy; most likely to occur in a chronic alcoholic patient with poor dietary intake)

Ascorbic acid deficiency (scurvy)

Nicotinic acid deficiency (pellagra characterized by mental confusion and peripheral neuropathy; may occur in chronic alcohol abuse patient or in the presence of a carcinoid tumor)

Vitamin A deficiency (conjunctival drying and anemia)

Vitamin D deficiency (thoracic kyphosis)

Vitamin K deficiency (prolonged antibiotic therapy or absence of bile salts; prolonged prothrombin time)

XV. DISORDERS RELATED TO VITAMIN IMBALANCE
(Table 23-13)

CHAPTER 24

Anemia

Anemia, like fever, is a sign of disease manifesting clinically as a numerical deficiency of erythrocytes (RBCs) (see Stoelting RK, Dierdorf SF. Anemia. In: Anesthesia and Co-Existing Disease. 3rd Ed. New York. Churchill Livingstone, 1993). The most important adverse effect of anemia is decreased tissue oxygen delivery owing to the associated decrease in arterial content of oxygen (CaO_2). Compensation for decreased CaO_2 is accomplished by a rightward shift of the oxyhemoglobin dissociation curve and an increase in cardiac output (Fig. 24-1).

I. IRON DEFICIENCY ANEMIA

A. Nutritional deficiency of iron is a cause of anemia only in infants and small children.

B. In adults, iron deficiency anemia can only reflect depletion of iron stores owing to chronic blood loss (gastrointestinal tract, menstruation). Parturients are susceptible to the development of iron deficiency anemia because of increased RBC mass during gestation and the needs of the fetus for iron.

C. **Treatment** of iron deficiency anemia is with iron salts administered orally. In the future, erythropoietin may be used to improve the hematocrit before elective surgery.

D. Management of Anesthesia

1. A **minimum acceptable hemoglobin concentration** (10 $g \cdot dl^{-1}$ frequently quoted) cannot be recommended on the basis of available evidence.

2. Transfusion of RBCs is intended only to increase oxygen carrying capacity. The decision to transfuse preoperatively must be individualized and take into account several factors (Table 24-1).

3. Intraoperative changes that could further interfere with tissue oxygen delivery (decreases in cardiac output, leftward shift of the oxyhemoglobin dissociation curve as due to respiratory alkalosis, PaO_2 <100 mmHg) are avoided (Fig. 24-1).

   a. Any decrease in tissue oxygen delivery during anesthesia may be offset by decreased tissue oxygen

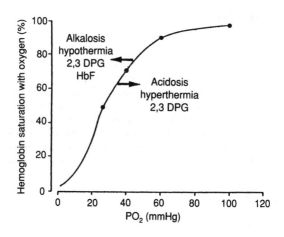

Fig. 24-1. *The oxyhemoglobin dissociation curve describes the relationship between saturation of hemoglobin with oxygen and the PO_2.*

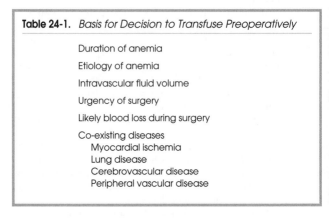

Table 24-1. *Basis for Decision to Transfuse Preoperatively*

Duration of anemia

Etiology of anemia

Intravascular fluid volume

Urgency of surgery

Likely blood loss during surgery

Co-existing diseases
Myocardial ischemia
Lung disease
Cerebrovascular disease
Peripheral vascular disease

requirements due to hypothermia or depressant effects of anesthetic drugs.

    b. Blood loss is promptly replaced when there is co-existing anemia, especially if the hemoglobin concentration acutely decreases to <7 g·dl^{-1}.

4. Postoperatively, it is important to minimize shivering or increases in body temperature that could increase tissue oxygen requirements.

II. **ANEMIA OF CHRONIC DISEASE** (Table 24-2). This form of anemia is usually mild, rarely requiring treatment with blood transfusions (iron is not effective).

III. **THALASSEMIA** is an inherited disorder of hemoglobin synthesis that results in anemia that may require treatment with blood transfusions.

IV. **ACUTE BLOOD LOSS** (Table 24-3)
   A. **Hematocrit** may not reflect anemia due to acute blood loss, since physiologic mechanisms for restoring plasma volume operate slowly.
   B. **Hemorrhagic Shock**

Table 24-2. *Chronic Diseases Associated With Anemia*

Infections

Cancer

Connective tissue disorders

Acquired immunodeficiency syndrome

Alcoholic liver disease

Renal failure

Diabetes mellitus

Table 24-3. *Clinical Signs Associated With Acute Blood Loss*

Blood Volume Lost (%)	Signs
10	None
20–30	Orthostatic hypotension Tachycardia
40	Tachycardia Hypotension Tachypnea Diaphoresis

1. Treatment is with infusion of whole blood and crystalloid solutions.
   a. Invasive monitoring is often necessary to guide the adequacy of intravascular fluid volume replacement and to evaluate the response to inotropes (vasopressors are used sparingly).
   b. Persistent metabolic acidosis probably reflects the continued presence of hypovolemia and inadequate tissue oxygen delivery.
2. **Management of anesthesia.** Induction and maintenance of anesthesia in the presence of hemorrhagic shock requires invasive monitoring and often includes the administration of ketamine.

V. **APLASTIC ANEMIA** is most often due to destruction of bone marrow stem cells by cancer chemotherapeutic drugs resulting in pancytopenia.

   A. **Fanconi syndrome** is congenital aplastic anemia plus numerous associated anomalies (microcephaly, short stature, cleft palate, cardiac defects).
   B. **Diamond-Blackfan syndrome** is a form of pure erythrocyte aplasia treated with RBCs and corticosteroids.
   C. **Management of anesthesia** in the presence of aplastic anemia includes consideration of drugs used in treatment, susceptibility to infection, and occurrence of hemorrhage with minor trauma (tracheal intubation must be atraumatic).

VI. **MEGALOBLASTIC ANEMIA** is most often due to deficiencies of vitamin B_{12} or folic acid. **Management of anesthesia** includes consideration of the likely presence of peripheral neuropathy and possible presence of liver disease due to alcoholism.

VII. **HEMOLYTIC ANEMIAS** (Table 24-4)

   A. **Sickle cell disease** reflects the presence of an inherited defect in hemoglobin structure (hemoglobin S), as confirmed by hemoglobin electrophoretic studies.
   B. **Sickle cell trait** is the heterozygous manifestation of sickle cell disease present as an asymptomatic disease in 8% to 10% of African Americans.

Table 24-4. *Hemolytic Anemias*

> Hereditary spherocytosis (cholecystitis is common; splenectomy if anemia is severe)
>
> Paroxysmal nocturnal hemoglobinuria (thrombosis is a hazard)
>
> Glucose 6-phosphate dehydrogenase deficiency (triggered by drugs; hemolysis and jaundice in the postoperative period is suggestive)
>
> Pyruvate kinase deficiency
>
> Immune hemolytic anemia (diagnosed by Coombs test; may be due to drugs, diseases, or sensitization of erythrocytes)
>
> Cold hemagglutinin disease (see Table 29-6)
>
> Sickle cell disease
>
> Methemoglobinemia (diagnosed by presence of cyanosis in presence of normal PaO_2 and low measured SaO_2; pulse oximeter reads 85%; treatment is methylene blue)
>
> Sulfhemoglobinemia

Table 24-5. *Signs and Symptoms of Sickle Cell Anemia*

> Anemia (hemoglobin 5–10 $g \cdot dl^{-1}$)
>
> Jaundice
>
> Excruciating musculoskeletal pain
>
> Cor pulmonale (pulmonary emboli)
>
> Increased alveolar-to-arterial difference for oxygen

C. **Sickle cell anemia** is the homozygous manifestation of sickle cell disease present in 0.2% of African Americans as evidenced by **chronic hemolysis** and acute episodic **vaso-occlusive crises** that cause organ failure.
1. **Signs and Symptoms** (Table 24-5)
2. **Treatment** may include neuraxial analgesia.
3. **Management of anesthesia** is not likely to be altered by the presence of sickle cell trait, whereas the presence of sickle cell anemia introduces unique considerations (Table 24-6).

Table 24-6. *Management of Anesthesia in the Presence of Sickle Cell Anemia*

Preoperative Preparation
Correct infection
Hydration
Consider transfusion (goal is hemoglobin A concentration near 50% and hematocrit near 35%)

Intraoperative Management
Avoid acidosis (hypoventilation)
Prevent circulatory stasis (body positioning, tourniquets, hypovolemia, hypotension)
Maintain normothermia
Maintain optimal oxygenation (supplemental oxygen during regional anesthesia)

Postoperative Care
Supplemental oxygen
Maintain normovolemia
Maintain normothermia

VIII. LEUKOCYTES (Table 24-7)

Table 24-7. *Leukocytes and Clinical Importance*

	Range (cells·mm^{-3})	Total (%)	Physiologic Significance
All leukocytes	4300–10,000	100	
Neutrophils	1800–7200	55	Defense against bacterial infection
Lymphocytes	1500–4000	36	Production of immunoglobulins
Eosinophils	0–700	2	Response to allergic reactions and fungal infections
Basophils	0–150	1	Release chemical mediators
Monocytes	200–900	6	Modify immune response, phagocytosis

Table 24-8. *Causes of Polycythemia*

Secretion of erythropoietin

Decrease in PaO_2 <60 mmHg (ascent to altitude, cardiopulmonary disease)

Cigarette smoking (carboxyhemoglobin results in tissue hypoxia that stimulates secretion of erythropoietin)

IX. POLYCYTHEMIA is present when the hematocrit is >55% (Table 24-8). Adverse effects of polycythemia are due principally to increased viscosity of the blood.

CHAPTER 25

Coagulation Disorders

Coagulation disorders may be hereditary or acquired (Table 25-1) (see Stoelting RK, Dierdorf SF. Coagulation disorders. In: Anesthesia and Co-Existing Disease. 3rd Ed. New York. Churchill Livingstone, 1993).

I. PHYSIOLOGY OF COAGULATION

A. Arrest of bleeding from a damaged blood vessel depends on (1) vasoconstriction at the site of injury, (2) formation of a platelet plug at the site of injury, and (3) activation of the clotting cascade (Fig. 25-1).

B. All the plasma procoagulants except von Willebrand factor (vWF) are synthesized in the liver (Table 25-2).

II. PREOPERATIVE EVALUATION (Table 25-3)

III. HEREDITARY COAGULATION DISORDERS are usually due to the absence or decreased presence of a single procoagulant.

A. **Hemophilia A** is an X-linked recessive disorder affecting males that is due to a defective or deficient factor VIII:C molecule.

1. A useful screening test is the partial thromboplastin time (PTT), which is prolonged in all but those with mild disease.

2. **Preoperative preparation** is intended to establish a factor VIII plasma concentration that will ensure hemostasis during the perioperative period (cryoprecipitate, desmopressin) (Table 25-4).

3. **Management of Anesthesia** (Table 25-5)

B. **Hemophilia B** is an X-linked genetic disorder caused by a defective or deficient factor IX molecule.

C. **von Willebrand's disease** affects both sexes and is due to deficient or defective amounts of vWF, which is necessary for the adherence of platelets to exposed endothelium.

1. Excessive bleeding from surgery or trauma is localized to the site of injury.

2. Treatment is with cryoprecipitate or desmopressin.

D. **Hereditary hemorrhagic telangiectasia** (Osler-Weber-

Table 25-1. *Categorization of Coagulation Disorders*

Hereditary
Hemophilia A
Hemophilia B
von Willebrand's disease
Afibrinogenemia
Factor V deficiency
Factor XIII deficiency
Hereditary hemorrhagic telangiectasia
Protein C deficiency
Antithrombin III deficiency

Acquired
Vitamin K deficiency
Drug-induced hemorrhage
Massive blood transfusion
Postcardiopulmonary bypass
Disseminated intravascular coagulation
Drug-induced platelet dysfunction
Idiopathic thrombocytopenic purpura
Thrombotic thrombocytopenic purpura
Catheter-induced thrombocytopenia

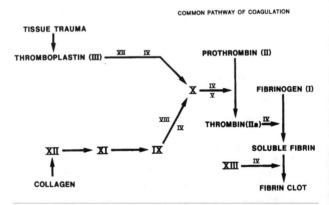

Fig. 25-1. *Schematic diagram of the events leading to activation of circulating procoagulants and culminating in the formation of a fibrin clot. Artificial division of the initial steps of the coagulation cascade into an intrinsic and extrinsic coagulation pathway is no longer recommended in view of the known interrelatioships between steps initiated by tissue trauma and/or collagen on the walls of damaged blood vessels.*

Table 25-2. *Plasma Procoagulants*

Factor	Synonym	Plasma Concentration ($\mu g \cdot ml^{-1}$)	Half-time (h)	Minimal Level for Surgical Hemostasis (% of normal)	Stability on Storage in Whole Blood (4°C, 21 days)
I	Fibrinogen	2500–3500	95–120	50–100	No change
II	Prothrombin	100	65–90	20–40	No change
III	Thromboplastin	—	—	—	—
IV	Calcium	—	—	—	—
V	Proaccelerin	10	15–24	5–20	Half-time 7 days
VII	Proconvertin	0.5	4–6	10–20	No change
VIII	Antihemophilic factor	15	10–12	30	Half-time 7 days
IX	Christmas factor	3	18–30	20–25	No change
X	Stuart–Prower factor	10	40–60	10–20	No change
XI	Plasma thromboplastin antecedent	<5	45–60	20–30	Half-time 7 days
XII	Hageman factor	<5	50–70	0	No change
XIII	Fibrin-stabilizing factor	20	72–120	1–3	No change

Table 25-3. *Preoperative Evaluation of Coagulation*

History (hemostatic response to prior surgery)

Physical examination (petechiae, ecchymoses)

Laboratory tests (perform only when indicated)
Platelet function (no evidence that skin bleeding time parallels bleeding elsewhere in the body)
Prothrombin time (12–14 sec)
Partial thromboplastin time (25–35 sec)
Thrombin time (12–20 sec)
Thromboelastography (measures procoagulants and platelets)

Table 25-4. *Factor VIII Concentrations Necessary for Hemostasis*

	Factor VIII Concentration (% of normal)
Spontaneous hemorrhage	1–3
Moderate trauma	4–8
Hemarthrosis and deep skeletal muscle hemorrhage	10–15
Major surgery	>30

Table 25-5. *Management of Anesthesia in the Patient With Hemophilia A*

Oral preoperative medication

Regional anesthesia may be avoided because of hemorrhagic tendency

Tracheal intubation acceptable

Consider likely presence of transfusion-related diseases

External pressure effective for controlling hemorrhage

Rendu syndrome) is characterized by the development of arteriovenous fistulas, especially in the lungs (air embolism, arterial hypoxemia) and systemic circulation (high-output congestive heart failure).

1. **Epistaxis** is a common complaint.
2. **Management of anesthesia** must consider the possibility of hemorrhage from telangiectatic lesions that may be present in the oropharynx, trachea, and esophagus.

E. **Hypercoagulable States**

1. **Protein C deficiency** most often presents as recurrent thromboembolic disease (myocardial infarction, cerebral infarction, pulmonary embolism).
   a. Thrombosis may be initiated by events that accompany the perioperative period (endothelial damage, immobility, stasis of blood flow).
   b. Regional anesthetic techniques may be useful alternatives to general anesthesia.
2. **Antithrombin III deficiency** is associated with an increased incidence of thromboembolic disease and resistance to the anticoagulant effects of exogenously administered heparin. Acute treatment is with administration of a specific concentrate or fresh frozen plasma (FFP).

IV. ACQUIRED COAGULATION DISORDERS

A. **Vitamin K deficiency** manifests as a prolonged prothrombin time (PT) in the presence of a normal PTT. If active bleeding is present, the administration of FFP is rapidly effective.

B. **Drug-induced hemorrhage** may be due to heparin (prolonged PT and PTT; treat with protamine) or coumarin (prolonged PT; treat with FFP).

1. **Anticoagulation and Regional Anesthesia**
   a. The prospect of administering a spinal or epidural anesthetic to a patient who will subsequently receive heparin is a controversial issue based on the concern that a spinal or epidural hematoma may result, should a blood vessel be damaged during performance of the anesthetic (risk is remote based on large retrospective reviews).
   b. Postoperative neurologic deficits should arouse suspicion of hematoma formation.

2. **Regional anesthesia in the presence of anticoagulation** is selected based on the presumed benefits of the block relative to alternative techniques.

C. **Massive blood transfusion** (>10 units of blood and/or persistent volume deficit) can lead to a coagulation disorder characterized by diffuse microvascular bleeding (abnormal thrombelastograph and prolonged PT and PTT) (Fig. 25-2). There is no justification for prophylactic administration of platelets or FFP in the massively transfused patient.

D. **Postcardiopulmonary bypass** bleeding is most likely due to an acquired platelet function disorder.

E. **Disseminated intravascular coagulation (DIC)** is characterized by uncontrolled activation of the coagulation system with consumption of platelets and procoagulants. **Treatment** of DIC is correction of the provoking event (Table 25-6).

F. **Drug-induced platelet dysfunction** (aspirin, nonsteroidal anti-inflammatory drugs) reflects irreversible interference with platelet release of adenosine diphosphate (ADP) and subsequent platelet aggregation.

1. **Treatment** is transfusion of platelets that can release ADP.

2. **Aspirin and elective surgery** do not seem to be associated with increased perioperative blood loss or with an increased incidence of neurologic complications when spinal or epidural anesthesia is performed.

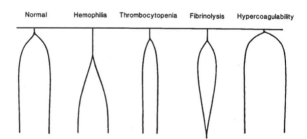

| Normal | Hemophilia | Thrombocytopenia | Fibrinolysis | Hypercoagulability |

Fig. 25-2. *Schematic depiction of coagulopathy, as reflected by the thrombelastograph.*

Table 25-6. *Causes of Disseminated Intravascular Coagulation*

Crush injury

Hemorrhagic shock

Severe intracranial damage

Extensive surgery

Retained placenta

Burn injury

Hemolytic transfusion reaction

Malignant hyperthermia

Prolonged cardiopulmonary bypass

Gram-negative sepsis

Tumor products

Snake bites

G. Idiopathic thrombocytopenic purpura (ITP) is characterized by thrombocytopenia (often <50,000 cells·mm^{-3}) and evidence of petechiae formation.
   1. **Treatment** is initially with a corticosteroid.
   2. **Management of anesthesia** includes platelet transfusions, minimization of trauma to the airway during direct laryngoscopy for tracheal intubation, and avoidance of regional anesthesia.
H. Catheter-induced thrombocytopenia may reflect thrombus formation on the catheter with associated consumption of platelets.

V. TRANSFUSION THERAPY

   A. Component Therapy (Table 25-7)
   B. Complications of Blood Transfusion (Table 25-8)

Table 25-7. *Component Therapy*

Packed erythrocytes (only indication is to increase oxygen-carrying capacity of blood; 1 unit will increase hemoglobin concentration about 1 g·dl^{-1})

(Continues)

Table 25-7. *Component Therapy* (Continued)

Platelets (only indication is documented thrombocytopenia or platelet dysfunction; 1 unit will increase platelet count about 5000 cells•mm^{-3} before invasive elective surgery)

Fresh frozen plasma (only indication is a documented procoagulant deficiency)

Cryoprecipitate (high concentrations of factor VIII and fibrinogen)

Plasma volume expanders
　Albumin
　Plasma protein fraction
　Dextran
　Hetastarch
　Crystalloid (need 3–4 ml for every 1 ml of estimated blood loss)

Table 25-8. *Complications of Blood Transfusions*

Transmission of viral diseases

Transfusion reactions
　Allergic (pruritus, urticaria, and increase in body temperature; treatment is diphenhydramine 0.5–1 mg•kg^{-1} IV)
　Febrile (temperature rarely exceeds 38°C; treatment is an antipyretic)
　Hemolytic (ABO incompatibility; manifests as hemolysis, hypotension, and disseminated intravascular coagulation)
　Delayed hemolytic (jaundice 10–14 days after administration of correctly cross-matched blood)

Metabolic abnormalities

Microaggregates

Immunosuppression

CHAPTER 26

Skin and Musculoskeletal Diseases

Skin and musculoskeletal diseases may influence the selection of anesthetic techniques and drugs administered in the perioperative period (see Stoelting RK, Dierdorf SF. Skin and musculoskeletal diseases. In: Anesthesia and Co-Existing Disease. 3rd Ed. New York. Churchill Livingstone, 1993).

I. **EPIDERMOLYSIS BULLOSA** is a rare hereditary disorder of the skin characterized by bullae formation, especially when lateral shearing forces are applied to the skin.

    A. **Treatment** is symptomatic and often includes corticosteroids.

    B. **Management of Anesthesia** (Table 26-1)

II. **PEMPHIGUS** is a vesiculobullous disease that may involve the skin and mucous membranes (see section I and Table 26-1).

III. **PSORIASIS** is a common dermatologic disorder characterized by accelerated epidermal growth. It is often treated with topical corticosteroids. An inflammatory asymmetric arthropathy occurs in about 20% of patients.

IV. **MASTOCYTOSIS** is characterized by an abnormal proliferation of mast cells in the skin (urticaria pigmentosa) or viscera (systemic mastocytosis).

    A. **Signs and symptoms** reflect degranulation of mast cells and release of histamine, heparin, and prostaglandins into the systemic circulation.

    B. **Management of anesthesia** is usually uneventful. However, life-threatening anaphylactoid reactions are a possibility.

V. **COLD URTICARIA** in a highly sensitive patient may manifest as laryngeal edema and bronchospasm on exposure to cold.

VI. **ERYTHEMA MULTIFORME** may manifest as bullous lesions, often in association with drug-induced hypersensi-

Table 26-1. *Management of Anesthesia in the Presence of Epidermolysis Bullosa*

Avoid trauma to skin and mucous membranes (suture catheters or hold in place with gauze wrap).

Consider cortisol ointment application to face mask.

Minimize frictional trauma to orpharynx (lubricate laryngoscope blade).

Tracheal intubation is acceptable.

Increased incidence of porphyria may influence selection of drugs.

Succinylcholine is acceptable.

tivity. **Stevens-Johnson syndrome** is a multisystem manifestation (fever, tachycardia) of erythema multiforme.

VII. SCLERODERMA (progressive systemic sclerosis) is characterized by inflammation, vascular sclerosis, and fibrosis of the skin and viscera. The prognosis is poor. Corticosteroids are not recommended.

 A. **Signs and Symptoms** (Table 26-2)
 B. **Management of anesthesia** is influenced by the multiple organ systems likely to be involved by the progressive changes associated with this disease (Table 26-2).

VIII. PSEUDOXANTHOMA ELASTICUM is characterized by degeneration and calcification of elastic fibers leading to loss of visual acuity, gastrointestinal hemorrhage, hypertension, and ischemic heart disease.

IX. EHLERS-DANLOS SYNDROME is an inherited connective tissue disorder characterized by hypermobility of the joints and increased extensibility of the skin. **Management of anesthesia** may be influenced by other abnormalities associated with this syndrome (Table 26-3).

X. POLYMYOSITIS (dermatomyositis) is an inflammatory myopathy. Skeletal muscle weakness may lead to dysphagia, pulmonary aspiration, and pneumonia. Myocarditis and

Table 26-2. *Signs and Symptoms of Scleroderma*

Skin and Musculoskeletal System
    Flexion contractures (fingers, mouth)
    Proximal skeletal muscle weakness

Nervous System
    Nerve compression
    Trigeminal neuralgia

Cardiovascular System
    Dysrhythmias
    Conduction abnormalities
    Congestive heart failure

Lungs
    Pulmonary fibrosis
    Arterial hypoxemia

Kidneys
    Accelerated hypertension

Gastrointestinal Tract
    Dysphagia
    Hypomotility

Table 26-3. *Abnormalities Associated With Ehlers-Danlos Syndrome*

Bleeding tendency (avoid intramuscular injections and instrumentation of the nose and esophagus)

Pneumothorax

Mitral regurgitation

Cardiac conduction abnormalities

Unrecognized extravasation of intravenous fluids

occult cancer are often present. The possibility of an exaggerated response to nondepolarizing muscle relaxants and postoperative ventilatory insufficiency must be considered.

XI. **SYSTEMIC LUPUS ERYTHEMATOSUS** is a multisystem chronic inflammatory disease that may be drug induced (hydralazine, procainamide).

A. **Signs and symptoms** may be categorized as **articular** (symmetric arthritis) and **systemic** (pericarditis, pneumonia, glomerulonephritis, hepatitis, and skeletal muscle weakness).

  B. **Treatment** may include aspirin and corticosteroids.

  C. **Management of anesthesia** is influenced by drugs used in treatment and symptoms due to organ damage produced by the disease.

XII. **MUSCULAR DYSTROPHY** is a hereditary disease characterized by painless degeneration and atrophy of skeletal muscles, often in association with mental retardation (Table 26-4).

XIII. **MYOTONIC DYSTROPHY** is a hereditary disease of skeletal muscles characterized by persistent contracture of skeletal muscles in response to stimulation (not relieved by anesthesia or muscle relaxants) (Table 26-5).

XIV. **MYASTHENIA GRAVIS** is a chronic autoimmune disease involving the neuromuscular junction. This disease is characterized by weakness and rapid exhaustion of skeletal muscles with repetitive use, followed by partial recovery with rest.

  A. **Signs and symptoms** of myasthenia gravis are characterized by periods of exacerbation and remission (Table 26-6).

Table 26-4. *Classification and Characteristics of Muscular Dystrophy*

Pseudohypertrophic Muscular Dystrophy
  Congestive heart failure
  Recurrent pneumonia
  Kyphoscoliosis
  Hyperkalemia with succinylcholine
  Malignant hyperthermia susceptible(?)

Limb-Girdle Muscular Dystrophy (relatively benign disease)

Facioscapulohumeral Muscular Dystrophy (heart not involved)

Nemaline Rod Muscular Dystrophy
  Micrognathia
  Bulbar palsy

Table 26-5. *Classification and Characteristics of Myotonic Dystrophy*

Myotonic Dystrophica
    Cardiomyopathy
    Cardiac conduction disturbances (sudden death)
    Pulmonary aspiration
    Central sleep apnea
    Prolonged contraction in response to succinyl-choline
    Highly sensitive to drug-induced depression of ventilation

Myotonia Congenita (usually benign)

Paramyotonia (develops only on exposure to cold)

Table 26-6. *Signs and Symptoms of Myasthenia Gravis*

Ptosis and diplopia (most common initial symptoms)

Weakness of pharyngeal and laryngeal muscles (high risk of aspiration)

Asymmetric extremity skeletal muscle weakness (atrophy absent)

Cardiomyopathy

Hypothyroidism

B. Treatment (Table 26-7)
C. Management of Anesthesia (Table 26-8)

Table 26-7. *Treatment of Myasthenia Gravis*

Anticholinesterase drugs

Corticosteroids

Cyclosporine(?)

Plasmapheresis

Thymectomy (most likely elective operation)

Table 26-8. *Management of Anesthesia in the Presence of Myasthenia Gravis*

Preoperative Preparation
Avoid opioids
Inform patient that postoperative mechanical ventilation of the lungs is possible

Muscle Relaxants
Anticipate response that may be altered by disease or drugs used in treatment

Induction of Anesthesia
Short-acting intravenous drug
Consider tracheal intubation unassisted by muscle relaxants

Maintenance of Anesthesia
Volatile drug
Short- or intermediate-acting muscle relaxants

Postoperative Care
Recognize that skeletal muscle strength may decrease abruptly

XV. **MYASTHENIC SYNDROME** (Eaton-Lambert syndrome) is a disorder of neuromuscular transmission that resembles myasthenia gravis (Table 26-9).

Table 26-9. *Comparison of Myasthenic Syndrome and Myasthenia Gravis*

	Myasthenic Syndrome	Myasthenia Gravis
Manifestations	Proximal limb weakness (legs > arms)	Extraocular, bulbar, and facial muscle weakness
	Exercise improves strength	Fatigue with exercise
	Muscle pain common	Muscle pain uncommon
	Reflexes absent or decreased	Reflexes normal

(Continues)

Table 26-9. *Comparison of Myasthenic Syndrome and Myasthenia Gravis* (Continued)

	Myasthenic Syndrome	Myasthenia Gravis
Gender	Male > female	Female > male
Co-existing pathology	Small cell carcinoma of the lung	Thymoma
Response to muscle relaxants	Sensitive to succinylcholine and nondepolarizing muscle relaxants Poor response to anticholinesterase drugs	Resistant to succinylcholine Sensitive to nondepolarizing muscle relaxants Good response to anticholinesterase drugs

XVI. **FAMILIAL PERIODIC PARALYSIS** is characterized by intermittent but acute attacks of skeletal muscle weakness or paralysis. It usually spares only the muscles of respiration (bulbar musculature) (Table 26-10).

 A. **Management of anesthesia** is intended to avoid events that might precipitate skeletal muscle weakness (carbohydrate load, cold ambient temperature, potassium-losing diuretics).

 B. Frequent perioperative monitoring (every 15 to 60 minutes) of the plasma potassium concentration and aggressive intervention (potassium chloride up to 40 $mEq \cdot h^{-1}$ IV) is recommended.

XVII. **Prader-Willi syndrome** is characterized by skeletal muscle hypotonia, hypoglycemia, mental retardation, and the possible presence of micrognathia.

XVIII. **RHEUMATOID ARTHRITIS** is a chronic inflammatory disease characterized by symmetric polyarthropathy and significant systemic involvement (Table 26-11).

 A. **Management of anesthesia** must consider multiple organ involvement and side effects of drugs (aspirin and clot-

Table 26-10. *Clinical Features of Familial Periodic Paralysis*

Type	Plasma Potassium Concentration During Symptoms (mEq·L^{-1})	Precipitating Factors	Other Features
Hypokalemia	<3	Large glucose meals Strenuous exercise Glucose-insulin infusions Stress Hypothermia	Cardiac dysrhythmias Signs of hypokalemia on the electrocardiogram Sensitive to nondepolarizing muscle relaxants
Hyperkalemia	>5.5	Exercise Potassium infusions Metabolic acidosis Hypothermia	Sensitive to succinylcholine Skeletal muscle weakness may be localized to tongue and eyelids

Table 26-11. *Comparison of Rheumatoid Arthritis and Ankylosing Spondylitis*

	Rheumatoid Arthritis	Ankylosing Spondylitis
Family history	Rare	Common
Gender	Female (30–50 years old)	Male (20–30 years old)
Joint involvement	Symmetric polyarthropathy	Asymmetric oligoarthropathy
Sacroiliac involvement	No	Yes
Vertebral involvement	Cervical	Total (ascending)

(Continues)

Table 26-11. *Comparison of Rheumatoid Arthritis and Ankylosing Spondylitis* (Continued)

	Rheumatoid Arthritis	Ankylosing Spondylitis
Cricoarytenoid involvement	Common	No
Cardiac changes	Pericardial effusion Aortic regurgitation Cardiac conduction abnormalities Cardiac valve fibrosis Coronary artery arteritis	Cardiomegaly Aortic regurgitation Cardiac conduction abnormalities
Pulmonary changes	Pulmonary fibrosis Pleural effusion	Pulmonary fibrosis
Blood	Anemia	
Eyes	Keratoconjunctivitis sicca	Conjunctivitis Uveitis
Rheumatoid factor	Positive	Negative
HLA-B27	Negative	Positive
Treatment	Aspirin Corticosteroids Gold Surgery	

ting, corticosteroid supplementation) used in treatment (Table 26-11).

B. Airway evaluation includes consideration of the possible presence of atlantoaxial subluxation and determination of head movement or positions that can be tolerated by the awake patient without discomfort.

1. **Hoarseness or stridor** suggests involvement of the cricoarytenoid joints by arthritic changes.
2. Intubation of the trachea using a fiberoptic laryngoscope may be selected when preoperative evaluation suggests that direct visualization of the glottis may be difficult.

C. Preoperative pulmonary function studies and arterial

blood gases and pH may be indicated if severe lung disease is suspected.

D. The need for postoperative ventilatory support should be anticipated if severe restrictive lung disease is present preoperatively.

XIX. **SPONDYLARTHROPATHIES** are a group of non-rheumatic arthropathies that include ankylosing spondylitis (Marie-Strumpell disease), Reiter syndrome, juvenile chronic polyarthropathy, and enteropathic arthropathies (Table 26-11).

XX. **OSTEOARTHRITIS** is a degenerative process affecting articular cartilage that differs from rheumatoid arthritis in that there is minimal inflammatory reaction.

A. Degenerative changes are most significant in the middle to lower cervical spine and in the lower lumbar area.

B. **Treatment** includes aspirin and reconstructive joint surgery. Corticosteroids are not recommended.

XXI. **OSTEOPOROSIS** reflects the failure to mineralize adequately newly formed bone, especially in postmenopausal females.

XXII. **PAGET'S DISEASE** is characterized by osteoblastic and osteoclastic activity, resulting in abnormally thickened but weak bone.

XXIII. **OSTEOGENESIS IMPERFECTA** is an inherited defect of collagen production. It leads to brittle bones and associated fractures with trivial trauma (laryngoscopy), as well as the development of kyphoscoliosis.

XXIV. **MARFAN SYNDROME** is an inherited disorder of connective tissue and associated skeletal and cardiopulmonary abnormalities (Table 26-12). **Management of anesthesia** is influenced by cardiopulmonary abnormalities (prophylactic antibiotics, temporomandibular joint dislocation, avoid excessive pressor response to laryngoscopy).

XXV. **KYPHOSCOLIOSIS** is a deformity of the costovertebral skeletal structures characterized by an anterior flex-

---

Table 26-12. *Skeletal and Cardiovascular Abnormalities Associated With Marfan Syndrome*

> High arched palate
>
> Pectus excavatum
>
> Kyphoscoliosis
>
> Spontaneous pneumothorax
>
> Retinal detachment
>
> Mitral regurgitation (echocardiography)
>
> Dissection of the thoracic aorta (prophylactic beta antagonist therapy)

---

ion (kyphosis) and lateral curvature (scoliosis) of the vertebral column.

A. Signs and symptoms reflect restrictive lung disease (dyspnea, decreased vital capacity, poor cough reflex leading to recurrent pulmonary infections), and pulmonary hypertension.

B. Management of Anesthesia (Table 26-13)

Table 26-13. *Management of Anesthesia in the Presence of Kyphoscoliosis*

> Assess Physiologic Significance of Skeletal Deformity
> Pulmonary function tests
> Arterial blood gases
>
> Intraoperative Management
> Confirm adequacy of oxygenation
> Nitrous oxide may increase pulmonary vascular resistance
> Signs of malignant hyperthermia
>
> Surgery for Correction of Spinal Curvature
> Controlled hypotension
> Recognition of spinal cord injury (wake-up test, somatosensory evoked potentials)
>
> Postoperative Care
> Ensure adequate ventilation

XXVI. DEFORMITIES OF THE STERNUM characterized as pectus carinatum (outward protuberance) or pectus excavitum (inward concavity) produce psychological problems. Functional consequences are rare.

XXVII. ACHONDROPLASIA

   A. The predicted height for an achondroplastic male is 132 cm and for a female is 122 cm.

   B. Management of anesthesia in the achondroplastic dwarf may be influenced by predictable changes that accompany this disorder (Table 26-14).

XXVIII. HALLERMANN-STREIFF SYNDROME is characterized by oculomandibulodyscephaly and dwarfism. Direct laryngoscopy for tracheal intubation is both hazardous (brittle teeth, temporomandibular joint dislocation) and difficult.

XXIX. KLIPPEL-FEIL SYNDROME is characterized by shortness of the neck, cervical spine immobility, and occasionally the presence of micrognathia.

Table 26-14. *Characteristics of the Achondroplastic Dwarf That May Influence Management of Anesthesia*

Upper airway obstruction

Difficult exposure of glottic opening

Restrictive lung disease

Obstructive sleep apnea

Central sleep apnea

Pulmonary hypertension

Cor pulmonale

Hydrocephalus

Compressive spinal cord and nerve root syndromes
   Foramen magnum stenosis
   Odontoid hypoplasia with cervical instability
   Kyphoscoliosis

Thermal regulation dysfunction (hyperthermia)

CHAPTER 27

Infectious Diseases

Although infectious diseases are rarely the primary indications for surgery, not infrequently a co-existing infection (potentially transmissible) influences the management of a patient during the perioperative period (see Stoelting RK, Dierdorf SF. Infectious diseases. In: Anesthesia and Co-Existing Disease. 3rd Ed. New York. Churchill Livingstone, 1993). Infection is the most common cause of fever. Aspirin-like drugs (not physical cooling methods) are used to lower body temperature owing to an elevated hypothalamic setpoint.

I. ANTIBIOTICS

A. **Adverse reactions** to antibiotics include allergic reactions (penicillin versus cephalosporins; vancomycin) and altered neuromuscular conduction (aminoglycosides).

B. **Prophylactic antibiotics** (often cephalosporins) should be administered to coincide with bacterial inoculation. Prolongation of therapy beyond the first postoperative day probably provides no additional protection.

II. INFECTION DUE TO GRAM-POSITIVE BACTERIA (Table 27-1)

III. INFECTION DUE TO GRAM-NEGATIVE BACTERIA (Table 27-2). Fluid and electrolyte replacement is an important aspect of treatment.

IV. INFECTION DUE TO SPORE-FORMING ANAEROBES

A. **Clostridial myonecrosis** (gas gangrene) is a life-threatening infection that may be complicated by hypotension and renal failure.

1. **Treatment** consists of administration of an appropriate antibiotic and surgical débridement of infected tissues.

2. **Management of anesthesia** (Table 27-3)

B. **Tetanus** reflects elaboration of a neurotoxin that inhibits the release of acetylcholine at the neuromuscular junction while suppressing inhibitory internuncial neurons in the central nervous system.

Table 27-1. *Infections Due to Gram-Positive Bacteria*

Pneumococci
    Bacterial pneumonia
    Acute otitis media
    Penicillin or antibiotic with similar spectrum

Streptococci
    Group A
        Acute pharyngitis and tonsillitis (untreated may
           lead to rheumatic fever)
        Impetigo
        Cellulitis
        Penicillin or antibiotic with similar spectrum
    Group B
        Neonatal sepsis
    Group C
        Urinary tract infections
        Endocarditis

Staphylococci
    S. aureus
        Asympatomatic carriers
        Paronychia
        Surgical incision
        Contaminated food
    S. epidermidis
        Skin contaminants
        Bacteremia (intravenous catheters, prosthetic
           heart valves)

Table 27-2. *Infections Due to Gram-Negative Bacteria*

Salmonellosis
    Contaminated food
    Bacteremia (typhoid fever)

Shigellosis
    Diarrhea
    Dysentery

Cholera (hypotension and metabolic acidosis owing
to large fluid and electrolyte losses)

Escherichia coli diarrhea

Table 27-3. *Management of Anesthesia in the Presence of Clostridial Myonecrosis*

Consider multiple physiologic derangements
  Hypovolemia
  Anemia
  Renal failure

Theoretical concerns about use of nitrous oxide and succinylcholine are unsubstantiated

Electrocautery may be avoided (hydrogen gas)

Cross-infection unlikely

1. **Signs and Symptoms** (Table 27-4)
2. **Treatment** (Table 27-5)
3. **Management of anesthesia** often includes invasive monitoring and control of excessive sympathetic nervous system activity (volatile anesthetic, beta antagonist, lidocaine, nitroprusside).

Table 27-4. *Signs and Symptoms of Tetanus*

Trismus (especially of masseter muscles)

Laryngospasm

Inadequate ventilation due to spasm of intercostal muscles and diaphragm

Hyperthermia

Increased sympathetic nervous system activity (tachycardia, hypertension)

Table 27-5. *Treatment of Tetanus*

Control of skeletal muscle spasm (diazepam, nondepolarizing muscle relaxants)

Prevention of sympathetic nervous system hyperactivity (beta antagonist)

Support of ventilation of the lungs

Neutralization of circulating exotoxin (penicillin)

Surgical débridement

C. **Botulism** is characterized by acute and symmetric paralysis, owing to elaboration of a neurotoxin that interferes with presynaptic release of acetylcholine.

V. INFECTION DUE TO SPIROCHETES

A. **Syphilis** in its tertiary stage is characterized by destructive lesions in the nervous system (tabes dorsalis) and cardiovascular system (aortic regurgitation, ascending aortic aneurysm).

B. **Lyme disease** is characterized by multisystem involvement (cutaneous, fatigue, encephalopathy, neuropathy, heart block, arthritis) that undergoes remissions and exacerbations.

VI. INFECTION DUE TO MYCOBACTERIA is more likely to be present in Asian immigrants, elderly patients (particularly those in nursing homes), and those infected with human immunodeficiency virus (HIV). **Treatment** with isoniazid or rifampin may be associated with significant toxicity (hepatotoxicity, nephrotoxicity, neurotoxicity).

VII. SYSTEMIC MYCOTIC INFECTIONS (blastomycosis, coccidioidomycosis, histoplasmosis) are fungal infections characterized by pulmonary cavitary lesions that resemble tuberculosis.

VIII. INFECTION DUE TO *MYCOPLASMA* is manifested as nonproductive cough and pharyngitis (primary atypical pneumonia). Treatment is with erythromycin or tetracyclines.

IX. INFECTION DUE TO RICKETTSIAL ORGANISMS is manifested as Rocky Mountain spotted fever (rash, thrombocytopenia, abdominal pain, nonspecific ST changes) or Q fever (hepatosplenomegaly).

X. VIRAL INFECTIONS OF THE UPPER RESPIRATORY TRACT (Table 27-6)

A. These diseases are likely to be transmitted between patients and hospital personnel.

B. **Management of Anesthesia**

1. A common recommendation is to avoid anesthesia that

Table 27-6. *Viral Infections of the Upper Respiratory Tract*

Influenza virus (spread is via nasopharyngeal secretions of infected patients; self-limited unless complicated by bacterial infection or co-existing chronic pulmonary disease)

Rhinovirus (acute coryza; spread by contact with contaminated environmental surfaces or from skin of infected individuals)

Adenovirus (pharyngitis and conjunctivitis most common in children)

Respiratory syncytial virus (infant pneumonia and bronchiolitis)

Parainfluenza virus (laryngotracheobronchitis)

requires tracheal intubation in the patient with, or recovering from, a viral upper respiratory tract infection.

2. Airway hyperreactivity, bronchospasm, and laryngospasm are more frequent intraoperatively in the patient with a history of a recent upper respiratory tract infection.

XI. INFECTION DUE TO HERPES VIRUS (Table 27-7)

Table 27-7. *Infection due to Herpes Virus*

Herpes simplex virus type 1 (spread by oral secretions; whitlow)

Herpes simplex virus type 2 (genital transmission)

Varicella-zoster virus
    Varicella
    Herpes zoster (incidence increased in immunosuppressed patients)

Cytomegalovirus (heterophile-negative mononucleosis syndrome)

Epstein-Barr virus (heterophile-positive mononucleosis; hepatitis)

XII. ACQUIRED IMMUNODEFICIENCY SYNDROME

(AIDS) describes the occurrence of a life-threatening opportunistic infection and/or Kaposi sarcoma in a patient who demonstrates profound immunosuppression unrelated to drug therapy or known co-existing disease. The disease is caused by a retrovirus (HIV) that damages or destroys T lymphocytes, leading to cell-mediated immunodeficiency.

A. **Transmission** of HIV by routes other than sexual contact, transfusion of blood products, or communal intravenous drug use is virtually unknown.

1. There is no evidence of airborne transmission of HIV.

2. HIV is sensitive to common disinfectants and routine hospital sterilization techniques.

B. **Pathogenesis.** Antibodies are produced against HIV. They form the basis for most of the diagnostic tests for AIDS (HIV antibody positive) but offer little protection to the host against the development of the disease.

C. **Signs and symptoms** of AIDS reflect infectious and neurologic complications (Tables 27-8 and 27-9).

Table 27-8. *Infectious Complications of Acquired Immunodeficiency Syndrome*

Infecting Organism	Type of Infection
Bacteria	
Streptococcus	Pneumonia, disseminated infection
Hemophilus influenza type B	Pneumonia, disseminated infection
Salmonella	Gastroenteritis, disseminated infection
Virus	
Herpes simplex	Recurrent localized infection
Varicella-zoster	Localized disseminated infection
Cytomegalovirus	Pneumonia, retinitis, encephalitis, disseminated infection
Epstein-Barr	Lymphoproliferative disorders

(Continues)

Table 27-8. *Infectious Complications of Acquired Immunodeficiency Syndrome* (Continued)

Infecting Organism	Type of Infection
Fungus	
Candida albicans	Mucocutaneous infection, esophagitis, disseminated infection
Aspergillus	Necrotizing bronchopneumonia, disseminated infection
Cryptococcus	Meningitis, disseminated infection
Pneumocystis carinii	Pneumonia
Mycobacteria	Tuberculosis, disseminated infection

Table 27-9. *Neurologic Disorders Associated With Human Immunodeficiency Virus*

Disorder	Incidence (%)	Manifestations
Encephalitis	90	Memory loss Ataxia Seizures
Peripheral neuropathy	10–50	Paresthesias Weakness Sensory loss
Myelopathy	11–20	Spastic paresis Incontinence
Aseptic meningitis	5–10	Fever Headache Cranial nerve palsies

- **D. Treatment** is dependent on drug therapy, such as azidothymidine, which may produce anemia and granulocytopenia.
- **E. Management of anesthesia** assumes that all patients are potentially infected with HIV or other bloodborne pathogens (**barrier precautions**) (Table 27-10).

Table 27-10. *Universal Precautions to Prevent Transmission of Human Immunodeficiency Virus*

1. Blood and body fluid precautions should be used for all patients, recognizing that it is not possible to reliably identify infected patients.

2. Use barrier precautions to prevent skin and mucous membrane exposure to blood or body fluids that may contain blood.
   a. Wear gloves.
   b. Wear protective eye shields if droplets likely.
   c. Take care to prevent injury when handling sharp devices—do not recap needles.

3. Health care workers with exudative skin lesions should refrain from direct patient care.

4. Use equipment for cardipulmonary resuscitation that negates the need for mouth-to-mouth resuscitation.

(Adapted from Recommendations for Prevention of HIV Transmission in Health-Care Setting. MMWR 1987;36:2S, with permission.)

1. Disposable anesthetic equipment may be recommended in view of potential contamination with blood-contaminated secretions.
2. Laryngoscope blades and other nondisposable equipment that may come in contact with mucosal surfaces are thoroughly washed and sterilized.
3. Choice of anesthetic drugs, techniques, and monitors is influenced by accompanying systemic manifestations of AIDS and associated opportunistic infections (Tables 27-8 and 27-9).
4. Should a health care worker experience a needle stick from a patient with AIDS, it is recommended that serologic testing be conducted approximately every 6 weeks (most persons will convert in 1 to 3 months), recognizing that transmission by a single needle stick is unlikely.

XIII. **NOSOCOMIAL INFECTION** is an infection that occurs during the course of a hospital stay (pneumonia, surgical wound infection).

A. **Anesthesia equipment** as a source of cross-contamination between patients is cited as a reason to use disposable anesthetic equipment (validity of this recommendation is unproven).

B. Gram-negative bacteremia is often a reflection of nosocomial infection.

XIV. SEPTIC SHOCK can be divided into early (hyperdynamic) and late (hypovolemic) phases (Fig. 27-1).

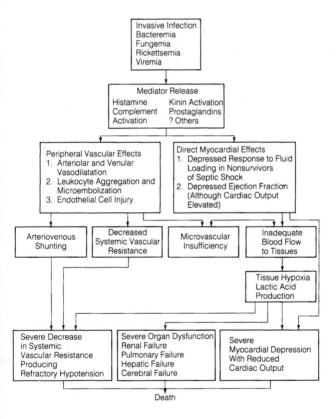

Fig. 27-1. *Flow diagram of the pathogenesis of septic shock in humans. (From Parker MM, Parrillo JE. Septic shock. Hemodynamics and pathogenesis. JAMA 1983;250:3324–7, with permission.)*

A. **Diagnosis** is suggested by the development of hypotension in the presence of peripheral vasodilation and oliguria, especially after procedures on the genitourinary tract.

B. **Treatment** consists of intravenous administration of antibiotics and repletion of intravascular fluid volume (guide by measurement of cardiac filling pressures and urine output).

   1. Dopamine is an effective inotropic drug when pharmacologic support of both blood pressure and renal function is necessary.

   2. Immunologic therapy uses monoclonal antibodies.

   3. Corticosteroids are not of proven efficacy in the treatment of septic shock.

C. Ketamine is an acceptable drug for induction of anesthesia in the patient experiencing septic shock.

XV. **INFECTIVE ENDOCARDITIS** is a microbial infection that implants on a heart valve or wall of the endocardium after transient bacteremia, especially in the presence of co-existing congenital heart disease. **Antibiotic prophylaxis** is recommended in susceptible patients when surgical procedures associated with bacteremia are planned (Table 27-11).

Table 27-11. *Procedures in Susceptible Patients for Which Antibiotic Prophylaxis Is Recommended*

Dental operations associated with gingival bleeding

Operations or procedures performed on the respiratory tract associated with disruption of the respiratory mucosa
   Tonsillectomy and adenoidectomy
   Nasotracheal intubation
   Bronchoscopy

Instrumentation of the gastrointestinal tract or genitourinary tract

Cardiac surgery

Noncardiac surgery in the patient with a prosthetic vascular graft or heart valve

Operations on infected tissues

XVI. **INFECTION OF THE CENTRAL NERVOUS SYS-TEM** may cause space-occupying lesions (abscess), evident on computed tomography or magnetic resonance imaging.

XVII. **BACTERIAL INFECTIONS OF THE UPPER RESPIRATORY TRACT** frequently follow processes (viral infections) that impair normal host-defense mechanisms (Table 27-12).

XVIII. **PULMONARY PARENCHYMAL INFECTION** most often follows processes (viral infections) that impair host-defense mechanisms manifesting as **bacterial pneumonia** (abrupt temperature elevation, arterial hypoxemia) or a **lung abscess** (alcoholism and poor dental hygiene are frequently present).

XIX. **INTRA-ABDOMINAL INFECTION** may manifest as **peritonitis** or **subphrenic** abscess (unexplained fever in a patient who has recently undergone intra-abdominal surgery).

Table 27-12. *Bacterial Infections of the Upper Respiratory Tract*

Acute sinusitis (intracranial extension a remote risk)

Acute otitis media (tympanoplasty tubes when recurrent infection; nitrous oxide may be avoided in presence of eustachian tube edema)

Pharyngitis (usually viral etiology; throat culture only way to distinguish clinically between streptococcal and viral pharyngitis)

Peritonsillar abscess (antibiotics and needle aspiration)

Retropharyngeal infection (upper airway obstruction possible)

Ludwig's angina (upper airway obstruction; tracheal intubation may not be possible)

Acute epiglottitis (see Chapter 32)

XX. **URINARY TRACT INFECTION** is the most common of all bacterial infections affecting humans, typically manifesting as dysuria and frequency.

XXI. **FEVER OF UNDETERMINED ORIGIN** is usually due to infection, neoplasm, or a connective tissue disorder.

XXII. **MUCOCUTANEOUS LYMPH NODE SYNDROME** (Kawasaki disease) is an acute febrile illness of children that may be associated with sudden death attributable to cardiac dysrhythmias or myocardial infarction (vasculitis and aneurysms of the coronary arteries).

XXIII. **INFECTION IN THE IMMUNOSUPPRESSED HOST** is a principal cause of morbidity and mortality.

A. Pneumonia is the most common cause of death in an immunosuppressed patient. A potentially fatal bacteremia may be associated with a trivial-appearing pulmonary infiltrate on a chest radiograph.

B. **Fungal infection,** especially **candidiasis** and *Pneumocystis carinii* (pneumonia that presents as a sudden onset of fever, tachypnea, progressive dyspnea, and arterial hypoxemia), is a common problem in the immunosuppressed host. A patient with *Pneumocystis* pneumonia may require supplemental oxygen and positive end-expiratory pressure to maintain acceptable arterial oxygenation.

CHAPTER 28

Cancer

Cancer is the second most frequent cause of death in the United States, being exceeded as a cause of mortality only by heart disease (see Stoelting RK, Dierdorf SF. Cancer. In: Anesthesia and Co-Existing Disease. 3rd Ed. New York. Churchill Livingstone, 1993). One of three Americans develops cancer, and one in five dies of it. Genes are involved in carcinogenesis by virtue of inheritance of traits that predispose to cancer (altered metabolism of potentially carcinogenic components, decreased level of immune system function) or by virtue of mutation of a normal cell gene to an **onco-gene.** Stimulation of oncogene formation by carcinogens (tobacco is the most frequent carcinogen) is estimated to be responsible for 80% of cancers in the United States.

I. DIAGNOSIS (Table 28-1)

II. TREATMENT (Table 28-2)

III. IMMUNOLOGY OF CANCER CELLS

  A. Tumor cells are antigenetically different from normal cells and may therefore elicit immune reactions similar to those that cause rejection of histoincompatible allografts.

  1. Antigens that are present in cancer cells but not in normal cells are designated **tumor-specific antigens.**

  2. Antigens that are present in cancer cells and in normal cells (concentration greater in tumor cells) are designated **tumor-associated antigens.**

  3. Antibodies to tumor-associated antigens can be used for the immunodiagnosis of cancer.

  B. Most spontaneously occurring tumors appear to be weakly antigenic.

IV. PATHOPHYSIOLOGIC DISTURBANCES (Table 28-3)

  A. Neuromuscular abnormalities manifesting as skeletal muscle weakness (myasthenic syndrome) may be associated with prolonged responses to muscle relaxants.

  B. Ectopic hormone production by tumors results in predictable physiologic effects (Table 28-4).

Table 28-1. *Diagnosis of Cancer*

Aspiration cytology

Biopsy (needle, incisional, excisional)

Monoclonal antibodies (recognize antigens for specific cancers, such as prostate, lung, breast, ovary)

Imaging techniques (computed tomography, magnetic resonance imaging)

Table 28-2. *Treatment of Cancer*

Chemotherapy (side effects may influence management of anesthesia)

Radiation

Surgery (removal of entire tumor or to decrease tumor mass, removal of metastases)

Bone marrow transplantation

Palliative and rehabilitative (may require surgery)

Pain relief

Table 28-3. *Pathophysiologic Manifestations of Cancer*

Fever	Tumor lysis syndrome
Anorexia	Adrenal insufficiency
Weight loss	Nephrotic syndrome
Anemia	Ureteral obstruction
Thrombocytopenia	Pulmonary osteoarthropathy
Coagulopathies	Pericardial effusion
Neuromuscular abnormalities	Pericardial tamponade
Ectopic hormone production	Superior vena cava obstruction
Hypercalcemia	Spinal cord compression
Hyperuricemia	Brain metastases

C. **Hypercalcemia** in the patient with cancer (lethargy, coma, polyuria) reflects osteolytic activity from bone metastases or ectopic hormonal activity.

Table 28-4. *Ectopic Hormone Production*

Hormone	Associated Cancer	Manifestations
Adrenocorticotropic hormone	Lung (small cell) Thyroid (medullary) Thymoma Carcinoid Non-beta islet cell of pancreas	Cushing syndrome
Antidiuretic hormone	Lung (small cell) Pancreas Lymphomas	Water intoxication
Gonadotropin	Lung (large cell) Ovary Adrenal	Gynecomastia Precocious puberty
Melanocyte stimulating hormone	Lung (small cell)	Hyperpigmentation
Parathyroid hormone	Renal Lung (squamous) Pancreas Ovary	Hyperparathyroidism
Thyroid stimulating hormone	Choriocarcinoma Testicular (embryonal)	Hyperthyroidism
Thyrocalcitonin	Thyroid (medullary)	Hypocalcemia
Insulin	Retroperitoneal tumors	Hypoglycemia

D. Acute Respiratory Complications

1. The acute onset of dyspnea may reflect extension of the tumor or effects of chemotherapy.
2. **Bleomycin-induced** interstitial pneumonitis and fibrosis is the most commonly encountered pulmonary complication of chemotherapy (Table 28-5).

E. Acute Cardiac Complications (Table 28-6)

F. Superior Vena Cava Obstruction (Table 28-7)

1. Treatment consists of prompt radiation or chemotherapy to reduce the size of the tumor, thereby relieving venous and airway obstruction.
2. Bronchoscopy and mediastinoscopy to obtain a tissue diagnosis can be hazardous, especially in the presence

Table 28-5. *Signs and Symptoms of Bleomycin-Induced Interstitial Pneumonitis*

Nonproductive cough

Dyspnea

Tachypnea

Fever

Altered diffusion capacity for carbon monoxide

Increased alveolar-to-arterial difference for oxygen

Radiographic evidence of diffuse pulmonary infiltrates

Table 28-6. *Cardiac Complications Related to Cancer*

Pericardial effusion (most common cause of electrical alternans)

Cardiac tamponade (most likely in assocciation with pericardial effusion due to carcinoma of the lung)

Atrial fibrillation

Cardiomyopathy (patients treated with doxorubicin or daunorubicin)
 Refractory congestive heart failure
 Cardiomegaly

Table 28-7. *Signs and Symptoms of the Superior Vena Cava Syndrome*

Venous engorgement (especially jugular veins and arm veins)

Dyspnea

Airway obstruction

Hoarseness (edema of vocal cords)

Increased intracranial pressure

of co-existing airway obstruction and increased pressure in the mediastinal veins.

G. **Spinal Cord Compression**

1. Pain, skeletal muscle weakness, sensory loss, and auto-

nomic nervous system dysfunction reflect the presence of a metastatic lesion into the epidural space.

2. Once total paralysis has developed, results of surgical laminectomy or radiation to decompress the spinal cord are equally poor.

V. MANAGEMENT OF ANESTHESIA

A. Preoperative evaluation of the patient with cancer requires a consideration of the possible known side effects of the disease (Table 28-3) and an understanding of the adverse effects evoked by cancer chemotherapeutic drugs (Table 28-8).

B. Clinical tests to detect preoperatively any side effects related to treatment with chemotherapeutic drugs may be useful (Table 28-9).

1. Bleomycin-treated patients may be vulnerable to interstitial pulmonary edema (consider use of colloid solutions, titration of delivered oxygen concentration, and need for postoperative support of ventilation).

2. Depressant effects of anesthetic drugs on myocardial contractility may be enhanced in the patient with drug-induced cardiac toxicity.

3. Signs of central nervous system depression, autonomic nervous system dysfunction, and peripheral neuropathies should be sought in the preoperative evaluation.

4. The presence of renal or hepatic dysfunction may influence the choice of anesthetic drug and muscle relaxant.

C. Preoperatively, correction of nutrient deficiencies, anemia, coagulopathy, and electrolyte abnormalities may be required.

D. Attention to aseptic technique is important, as immunosuppression occurs with most chemotherapeutic drugs.

VI. COMMON CANCERS ENCOUNTERED IN CLINICAL PRACTICE

A. **Carcinoma of the Lung**

1. This disease is categorized as squamous cell carcinoma, adenocarcinoma, large cell carcinoma, and small cell carcinoma (Table 28-10).

2. **Management of anesthesia** in the patient with carcino-

Table 28-8. *Adverse Side Effects Produced by Cancer Chemotherapeutic Drugs*

	Immuno-suppression	Thrombo-cytopenia	Leuko-penia	Anemia	Cardiac Toxicity	Pulm-onary Toxicity	Renal Toxicity
Alkylating agents							
Bulsulfan (Myleran)	+	+++	+++	+++		++	++
Chlorambucil (Leukeran)	+	++	++	++		+	
Cyclopho-sphamide (Cytoxan)	++++	+	++	+		+	+
Melphalan (Alkeran)	+	++	++	++		+	
Thiotepa (Thiotepa)	+	+++	+++	+++		+	
Antimetabolites							
Methotrexate (Methotrexate)	+++	+++	+++	+++		+	++
6-Mercaptopu-rine (Purinethol)	+++	++	++	++			++
Thioguanine (Thioguanine)	+++	+	++	++			
5-Fluorouracil (Fluorouracil)	++++	+++	+++	+++			
Plant alkaloids							
Vinblastine (Velban)	++	+	+++	+			
Vincristine (Oncovin)	++	+	++	+			+
Antibiotics							
Doxorubicin (Adriamycin)		+	+++	++	+++		
Daunorubicin (Daunomycin)	+	++	+++	++	+++		

Hepatic Toxicity	CNS Toxicity	Peripheral Nervous System Toxicity	Autonomic Nervous System Toxicity	Stomatitis	Plasma Cholinesterase Inhibition	Other
				+	+	Adrenocortical-like effect (+) Hemolytic anemia (++)
+	+				+	Hemolytic anemia (++)
+				+	++	Hemolytic anemia (++) Hemorrhagic cystitis (+++)
					+	Inappropriate ADH secretion (+)
					++	Hemolytic anemia (++) Hemolytic anemia (++)
+				+++		
+++				+		
+++				+		
	+			+++		
		+	+	+		Inappropriate ADH secretion (+)
	+	++	++			
+				++		Red urine (+)
				++		Red urine (+)

Table 28-8. *Adverse Side Effects Produced by Cancer Chemotherapeutic Drugs* (Continued)

	Immuno-suppression	Thrombo-cytopenia	Leuko-penia	Anemia	Cardiac Toxicity	Pulm-onary Toxicity	Renal Toxicity
Antibiotics *(Cont'd)*							
Bleomycin (Blenoxane)		+	+	+		+++	
Mithramycin (Mithracin)	+	++++	++++	+++			++
Nitrosoureas							
Carmustine (BiCNU)		++	++	++		+	+
Lomustine (CeeNU)		+++	+++	++			
Enzymes							
L-Asparaginase (Elspar)	++	+	+	+			+

ADH, antidiuretic hormone; +, minimal; ++, mild; +++, moderate; ++++, marked.
(Adapted from Selvin BL. Cancer chemotherapy: Implications for the anesthesiologist. Anesth Analg 1981;60:425–34, with permission.)

ma of the lung includes preoperative consideration of tumor-induced effects (malnutrition, pneumonia, pain, ectopic endocrine effects, metastases to bone and brain) and evaluation of underlying cardiac and pulmonary function, especially if lung resection is planned.

3. Mediastinoscopy is a useful diagnostic procedure but has important potential complications associated with its use (Table 28-11).

B. Carcinoma of the Breast

1. Diagnosis of breast cancer is established by excisional biopsy, followed at a later time by a more definitive

Hepatic Toxicity	CNS Toxicity	Peripheral Nervous System Toxicity	Autonomic Nervous System Toxicity	Stomatitis	Plasma Choline-sterase Inhibition	Other
				+++		
++	+			+++		Coagulation defects (+++) Hypocalcemia (+) Hypokalemia (+)
			+			
+			+			
+++	+		+			Hemorrhagic pancreatitis (+) Coagulation defects (+)

surgical procedure designed to decrease tumor bulk and thus enhance the effectiveness of systemic therapy (chemotherapy, hormonal therapy) or radiation designed to eradicate occult micrometastases.

2. Metastases to bone are frequent, emphasizing the importance of a bone scan and measurement of the alkaline phosphatase concentration.

C. Carcinoma of the Colon

1. Presenting symptoms of colorectal cancer vary with the anatomic location of the lesion, ranging from anemia and fatigue (ascending colon) to abdominal cramping and obstruction (transverse colon).

Table 28-9. *Preoperative Tests in the Patient With Cancer*

Hematocrit

Platelet count

White blood cell count

Prothrombin time

Electrolytes

Renal function tests

Liver function tests

Blood glucose concentration

Arterial blood gases

Chest radiograph

Electrocardiogram

Table 28-10. *Pathophysiology of Lung Cancer*

Type	Incidence (%)	Most Common Site of Metasteses at Diagnosis	Five-Year Survival With Surgery (%)	Associated Syndromes
Squamous	30	Mediastinal nodes Brain Liver	30	Hypercalcemia
Adenocarcinoma	29	Mediastinal nodes Brain Bone	17	Osteoarthropathy
Large cell	16	Mediastinal nodes Bone Brain	15	Galoctorrhea Gynecomastia
Small cell	24	Mediastinal nodes Bone	5	Eaton-Lambert syndrome

(Continues)

Table 28-10. *Pathophysiology of Lung Cancer* (Continued)

Type	Incidence (%)	Most Common Site of Metasteses at Diagnosis	Five-Year Survival With Surgery (%)	Associated Syndromes
Small cell (cont'd)		Liver		Hyponatremia owing to SIADH Cushing syndrome Hypocalcemia

SIADH, syndrome of inappropriate antidiuretic hormone release.

Table 28-11. *Complications Associated With Mediastinoscopy*

Hemorrhage

Pneumothorax

Venous air embolism

Compression of right subclavian artery (erroneous diagnosis of cardiac arrest if monitoring pulse or blood pressure distal to this site)

Compression of right carotid artery (may be manifested as a postoperative neurologic deficit)

Bradycardia

  a. Colorectal cancer initially spreads to regional lymph nodes and then through the portal venous circulation to the liver, the most common site of metastasis.

  b. When the primary tumor is in the distal rectum, tumor cells may escape the portal venous system and spread via the paravertebral plexus to the lungs.

 2. Surgical resection offers the greatest potential for cure in the patient with invasive colorectal cancer.

 3. **Management of anesthesia** for surgical resection of colorectal cancer may be influenced by disease-induced anemia and the effects of metastases, as may be present in the liver or lungs.

a. Chronic large bowel obstruction probably does not increase the risk of aspiration on induction of anesthesia, although extreme abdominal distension could interfere with adequate ventilation and oxygenation.

b. Immunosuppression produced by transfused blood may be undesirable, suggesting the value of an anesthetic technique that lowers blood pressure and thus intraoperative blood loss.

D. Carcinoma of the Prostate

1. The plasma concentration of prostate-specific antigen is increased in the presence of prostate cancer.

2. Symptoms of metastatic disease include bone pain, weight loss, spinal cord compression, and acute renal failure secondary to bilateral hydronephrosis.

3. Carcinoma of the prostate confined to the gland is usually cured by surgical excision.

4. Treatment of metastatic disease is palliative, as prostate cancer is under the influence of androgen hormones.

VII. LESS COMMON CANCERS ENCOUNTERED IN CLINICAL PRACTICE (Table 28-12)

Table 28-12. *Less Common Cancers Encountered in Clinical Practice*

Head and neck cancer

Thyroid cancer

Esophageal cancer

Cardiac tumors

Gastric cancer (presenting features indistinguishable from benign peptic ulcer)

Liver cancer (cirrhosis often present)

Gallbladder cancer (discovered unexpectedly at cholecystectomy)

Pancreatic cancer

(Continues)

Table 28-12. *Less Common Cancers Encountered in Clinical Practice* (Continued)

Renal cell carcinoma (high-output congestive heart failure may develop)

Bladder cancer

Testicular cancer (common in young males; curable, even when distant metastases are present)

Carcinoma of the uterine cervix (in situ treated with a cone biopsy)

Carcinoma of the uterus

Carcinoma of the ovary

Cutaneous melanoma (incidence increasing faster than that of any other cancer)

Cancer of the bone (multiple myeloma, osteosarcoma, Ewing's tumor, chondrosarcoma)

Lymphoma

Leukemia
   Adult T cell leukemia (retrovirus termed T cell lymphotropic virus has been isolated from affected patients)
   Polycythemia vera (hyperviscosity of blood responsible for symptoms; treatment is phlebotomy)

A. Head and Neck Cancer
1. A history of excessive cigarette smoking and alcohol abuse is present in most patients.
2. The most common sites of metastases are lung, liver, and bone (hypercalcemia).
3. Preoperative nutritional therapy may be indicated.
4. Surgical treatment often uses laser technology.

B. Thyroid Cancer
1. This cancer may be associated with pheochromocytoma in an autosomal disorder known as multiple endocrine neoplasia type II.
2. Excessive secretion of adrenocorticotropic hormone by the tumor may lead to Cushing syndrome.

C. Esophageal Cancer
1. Dysphagia and weight loss are the initial symptoms of esophageal cancer in 90% of patients.

2. Palliation may include surgical placement of a feeding tube or a polyvinyl esophageal prosthesis.
3. The likelihood of underlying alcohol-induced liver disease, of chronic obstructive pulmonary disease from cigarette smoking, and of cross-tolerance with other anesthetic drugs are considerations in the anesthetic management of an affected patient.
   a. Weight loss often parallels a decrease in intravascular fluid volume, manifested as hypotension during induction and/or maintenance of anesthesia.
   b. Dysphagia may be associated with an increased risk of aspiration.

D. **Cardiac Tumors**
   1. **Metastatic cardiac tumor** is often manifested as a hemorrhagic pericardial effusion.
   2. **Primary benign cardiac tumor** (cardiac myxoma) is most often a pedunculated intracavitary space-occupying lesion (Table 28-13).
      a. A left atrial myxoma (most common site) may mimic mitral valve disease, with the development of pulmonary edema.
      b. A right atrial myxoma will be manifested as isolated tricuspid stenosis, dyspnea, and arterial hypoxemia.
      c. Symptoms of obstruction produced by a cardiac myxoma may be altered by changes in body position.
      d. A right atrial myxoma probably should discourage the placement of a right atrial or pulmonary artery catheter.

E. **Pancreatic Cancer**
   1. Pancreatic cancer, despite its low incidence, is the fourth most common cause of cancer-related mortality.

Table 28-13. *Findings Suggestive of a Cardiac Myxoma*

Refractory congestive heart failure

Unexplained cardiac rhythm disturbances

Syncope related to position change

Unexplained systemic or pulmonary emboli

Pulmonary hypertension of unknown cause

  2. Celiac plexus block with alcohol or phenol is the most effective intervention for the treatment of pain owing to pancreatic cancer.

   a. Complications of celiac plexus block include hypotension due to sympathetic nervous system denervation, especially in the chronically ill hypovolemic patient.

   b. Computed tomography may be used to confirm proper needle placement before any solution is injected to act on the celiac plexus.

F. Carcinoma of the Uterus

  1. This cancer is often associated with obesity, hypertension, and diabetes mellitus.

  2. The most common manifestation is vaginal bleeding in a menopausal or perimenopausal female.

G. Lymphoma

  1. The most useful diagnostic test in the patient with a suspected lymphoma is a lymph node biopsy.

  2. Hodgkin's disease is an example of a lymphoma manifested as cyclic increases in body temperature, anemia, weight loss, and superior vena cava obstruction from invasion of the mediastinum by tumor.

   a. Peripheral neuropathies and spinal cord compression may occur as a direct result of tumor growth.

   b. Bone marrow involvement is unusual in Hodgkin's disease but not in other lymphomas.

H. Leukemia

  1. Leukemia is the uncontrolled production of leukocytes owing to cancerous mutation of lymphogenous cells or myelogenous cells.

   a. Lymphocytic leukemias begin in the lymph nodes. They are named according to the type of hematopoietic cell that is primarily involved (acute lymphoblastic leukemia, chronic lymphocytic leukemia, adult T cell leukemia).

   b. Myeloid leukemias begin as cancerous production of myelogenous cells in bone marrow, with spread to extramedullary organs (acute myeloid leukemia, chronic myeloid leukemia, polycythemia vera).

  2. The principal difference between normal and leukemic cells is the ability of the latter to continue to divide. Thus, many tissues (especially the bone marrow, liver, and lymph nodes) are infiltrated or replaced.

    a. Anemia may be profound; fatal infection or hemorrhage (thrombocytopenia) reflects bone marrow failure.

    b. Use of nutrients by rapidly proliferating cancerous cells depletes amino acids, leading to patient fatigue and metabolic starvation of normal tissues.

  3. Treatment of leukemia is most often with chemotherapy intended to decrease the number of tumor cells. The goals are regression of organomegaly and improved bone marrow function.

    a. These drugs depress activity of bone marrow, such that hemorrhage and infection become the determinants of maximum acceptable doses.

    b. Destruction of tumor cells by chemotherapy produces a uric acid load that may result in urate nephropathy.

    c. Nutritional support of the patient undergoing chemotherapy may be necessary to prevent hypoalbuminemia and loss of immunocompetence.

  4. Bone marrow transplantation offers the opportunity for cure of otherwise fatal diseases, including refractory leukemia.

    a. **The recipient** must undergo a preoperative regimen (chemotherapy and total body radiation), designed to achieve functional **bone marrow ablation.**

    b. **Donor bone marrow** (up to 1500 ml) is harvested via multiple aspirations obtained from the posterior iliac spines and iliac crests, most often during gener-

---

Table 28-14. *Manifestations of Graft-versus-Host Disease*

    Oral ulceration and mucositis

    Esophageal ulceration

    Diarrhea with fluid and electrolyte loss

    Hepatitis with coagulopathy

    Pancytopenia and immunodeficiency

    Bronchiolitis obliterans

    Interstitial pneumonitis

    Pulmonary fibrosis

    Renal failure

al anesthesia (nitrous oxide may be avoided; volume of blood loss parallels the quantity of marrow harvested).

c. Preoperative complications in the bone marrow recipient reflect the need to ablate the bone marrow (gastrointestinal toxicity, pulmonary fibrosis, restrictive cardiomyopathy, infection), and side effects of chemotherapeutic drugs (Table 28-8).

d. **Graft-versus-host disease** is a life-threatening complication of bone marrow transplantation affecting multiple organ systems (Table 28-14).

CHAPTER 29

Disorders Related to Immune System Dysfunction

The immune system, which consists of a number of lymphoid organs (thymus, lymph nodes, tonsils, spleen), is responsible for protecting the individual from infection and recognizing foreign substances (see Stoelting RK, Dierdorf SF. Disorders related to immune system dysfunction. In: Anesthesia and Co-Existing Disease. 3rd Ed. New York. Churchill Livingstone, 1993). The immunologically active cells of the immune system are lymphocytes, characterized as B lymphocytes and T lymphocytes (Fig. 29-1).

I. HUMORAL IMMUNITY

A. Humoral immunity is mediated by B lymphocytes that differentiate into antibody-producing plasma cells when stimulated by an antigen.

B. Antibodies are a heterogeneous group of plasma proteins designated immunoglobulins (Ig) (Table 29-1).

II. CELLULAR IMMUNITY

A. Cellular immunity is mediated by T lymphocytes (helper and suppressor lymphocytes) that regulate antibody production by B lymphocytes.

B. Activity of helper T lymphocytes is balanced by suppressor T lymphocytes.

1. Autoimmune diseases may reflect an excessive immune response due to a defect in suppressor mechanisms (see section IX).

2. Immunodeficiency may result from an exaggerated suppressor response.

III. COMPLEMENT SYSTEM

A. The complement system, composed of 18 plasma proteins, serves as the principal humoral effector of immunologically induced inflammation.

B. Complement activation can be initiated by either the classical pathway (antigen-antibody interaction) or the alternative pathway (bacterial polysaccharides) (Fig. 29-2).

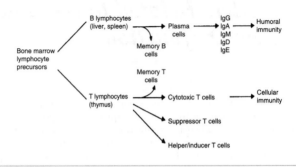

Fig. 29-1. *Schematic depiction of the immune system.*

Table 29-1. *Properties of Human Immunoglobulins*

	IgG	IgA	IgM	IgD	IgE
Location	Plasma Amniotic fluid	Plasma Saliva Tears	Plasma	Plasma	Plasma
Plasma concen- tration ($mg \cdot dl^{-1}$)	550–1900	60–333	45–145	0.3–30	Trace
Half-time (d)	23	6	5	3	2.5
Function	Immunity and defense against infection	Topical defense against infection	Lysis of bacterial cell walls	Not known	Anaphy- laxis

IV. ALLERGIC REACTIONS (Table 29-2)

A. **Anaphylaxis** is a life-threatening manifestation of an anti-gen-antibody interaction in which prior exposure of the host to a specific antigen (drug, food) has evoked produc-tion of antigen-specific IgE antibodies, rendering the host sensitized.

1. **Diagnosis** is suggested by the dramatic nature of the clinical manifestations (due to vasoactive mediators,

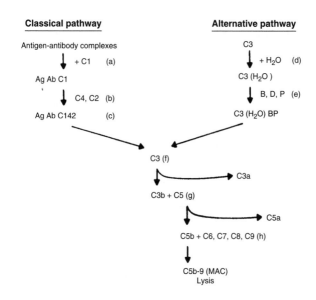

Fig. 29-2. *The complement system consists of the classical pathway and alternative pathway. (From Frank MM. Complement in the pathophysiology of human disease. N Engl J Med 1987;316:1525–30, with permission.)*

including histamine and leukotrienes released by degranulation of mast cells and basophils) in close temporal relationship to exposure to the antigen (usually within 5 to 10 minutes) (Table 29-3).

   a. Hypotension may be the only manifestation of anaphylaxis in the patient rendered unconscious by general anesthesia.

   b. It is conceivable that blockade of the innervation of the adrenal glands (spinal anesthesia, epidural anesthesia) could accentuate the symptoms of anaphylaxis by preventing the endogenous release of catecholamines.

2. Treatment is designed to reverse arterial hypoxemia, replace intravascular fluid, and inhibit further cellular degranulation with the release of vasoactive mediators (Table 29-4).

Table 29-2. *Examples of Allergic Reactions*

Anaphylaxis
Allergic Rhinitis (mimics viral respiratory tract infection)
Allergic Conjunctivitis
Allergic Asthma (see Chapter 14)
Food Allergy
Drug Allergy
    Muscle relaxants
    Barbiturates
    Propofol
    Local anesthetics
    Opioids
    Volatile anesthetics (especially halothane)
    Protamine
    Antibiotics
    Blood and plasma volume expanders
    Intravascular contrast media
    Vascular graft material
    Latex (natural rubber) containing medical
      devices)

Table 29-3. *Diagnosis of Anaphylaxis*

Rapid Onset of Symptoms
    Hypotension (may be accompanied by cardiac
      dysrhythmias and evidence of myocardial
      ischemia)
    Urticarial rash and pruritus
    Peripheral edema (reflects increased capillary per-
      meability and may account for 50% of the
      intravascular fluid volume)
    Laryngeal edema
    Bronchospasm
    Arterial hypoxemia
    Coagulopathy
Laboratory Tests
    Plasma immunoglobulin concentration
      (decreased early after reaction)
    Complement proteins
    Intradermal test (wheal and flare >4 mm in diame-
      ter)

(Continues)

Table 29-3. *Diagnosis of Anaphylaxis* (Continued)

> Laboratory Tests *(cont'd)*
> Radioallergosorbent test (RAST; commercially available antigens that will combine with antibodies in the patient's plasma)
> Plasma tryptase concentration (measure 15–60 minutes after the suspected allergic drug reaction; reflects mast cell degranulation)

Table 29-4. *Treatment of Anaphylaxis*

> Oxygen
> Intravenous fluids
> Epinephrine (10–100 µg IV)
> Diphenhydramine (50–100 mg IV)
> Albuterol (metered dose inhaler)
> Corticosteroids

    a. Early intervention with epinephrine (decreases release of vasoactive mediators, relaxes bronchial smooth muscle) is critical in reversing the life-threatening events characteristic of anaphylaxis.

    b. Beta-2 agonists such as albuterol have replaced aminophylline in the treatment of bronchospasm.

B. Drug Allergy

  1. Allergic reactions have been reported with virtually all drugs that may be injected during the administration of anesthesia (Table 29-2).

    a. The incidence of allergic drug reactions during anesthesia seems to be increasing, presumably reflecting the frequent administration of several drugs to the same patient, as well as cross-sensitivity between drugs.

    b. A history of allergy to specific drugs as elicited during the preoperative interview is helpful (a patient allergic to penicillin has a three- to fourfold greater risk of experiencing an allergic reaction to any drug). However, it must be appreciated that prior uneventful exposure to a drug does not eliminate the possibility of anaphylaxis on subsequent exposure.

2. **Muscle Relaxants**
   a. Drug-induced allergic reactions during the perioperative period are most often due to muscle relaxants.
   b. An estimated 50% of patients who experience an allergic reaction to one muscle relaxant will also be allergic to another muscle relaxant (all muscle relaxants contain one or more antigenic quaternary ammonium groups).

3. **Induction Drugs**
   a. There is often a history of prior uneventful exposure to the barbiturate induction drug that subsequently evokes an allergic reaction.
   b. Ketamine and benzodiazepines are unlikely to evoke allergic reactions.

4. **Local Anesthetics**
   a. It is important to differentiate an allergic reaction (urticaria, laryngeal edema, bronchospasm) from systemic toxicity (seizures, hypotension) or systemic absorption of epinephrine (tachycardia, hypertension).
   b. Ester local anesthetics, but not amide local anesthetics, are metabolized to the highly antigenic compound para-aminobenzoic acid (PABA). This accounts for the lack of cross-sensitivity between ester and amide local anesthetics.
   c. Local anesthetic solutions contain preservatives (methylparaben) that resemble PABA. Thus, anaphylaxis may be due to prior stimulation of antibody production by the preservative and not by the local anesthetic.

5. **Opioids**
   a. Anaphylaxis occurring after administration of opioids is rare, perhaps reflecting the similarity of these drugs to naturally present substances known as endorphins.
   b. Morphine, but not fentanyl or its related derivatives, may directly evoke the release of histamine from mast cells and basophils, producing an anaphylactoid reaction in a susceptible patient.

6. **Volatile Anesthetics** (see Chapter 18)
   a. Clinical manifestations of halothane hepatitis that suggest a drug-induced allergic reaction include eosinophilia, fever, rash, and prior exposure to halothane.

b. It is speculated that rare and possibly genetically susceptible individuals form antibodies in response to acetylation of liver proteins by an oxidative trifluoroacetyl halide metabolite of halothane.

c. A similar oxidative halide metabolite is also produced after exposure to enflurane and isoflurane. This emphasizes the possibility of cross-sensitivity between volatile anesthetics in susceptible patients.

7. Protamine

a. Anaphylactic reactions following administration of protamine may be more likely in the patient who is allergic to seafood and in the patient treated with a protamine-containing insulin preparation.

b. In susceptible patients, protamine may activate the complement pathway and evoke the release of thromboxane, leading to bronchoconstriction and pulmonary hypertension.

8. Antibiotics

a. Cross-sensitivity between penicillins and cephalosporins should prompt caution in the administration of the latter to a patient known to be allergic to penicillin.

b. Vancomycin is a potent stimulus to the release of histamine. It may produce life-threatening allergic reactions in susceptible patients, even when its administration rate is greatly slowed.

9. Blood and plasma volume expanders. Manifestations of an allergic reaction to blood range from pruritus, urticaria, and fever, to noncardiogenic pulmonary edema.

10. Latex-Containing Medical Devices

a. Unexplained cardiovascular collapse during anesthesia and surgery has been attributed to anaphylaxis triggered by latex (natural rubber).

b. Proteins in latex appear to be the source of antigens, especially if there is contact with mucous membranes (wheezing after inflating a toy balloon, rash or itching after wearing latex gloves).

c. Patients with spina bifida have an increased incidence of allergy to latex.

V. RESISTANCE TO INFECTION

A. Effects of anesthetics on resistance to infection are transient, reversible, and of minor importance, as compared with the prolonged immunosuppressive effects of cortisol and catecholamines released as part of the hormonal response to surgery.

- **B.** There is no evidence that the incidence of postoperative infection can be altered by the depth of anesthesia or by the techniques selected to produce anesthesia.

VI. RESISTANCE TO CANCER

- **A.** There is no evidence that short-term effects of anesthetic drugs are of any significance in the resistance of the host to cancer.
- **B.** As with infection, the more important concern is immuno-suppression produced by the hormonal response to surgical stimulation.

VII. DISORDERS OF THE IMMUNOGLOBULINS

- **A. X-Linked Agammaglobulinemia** (Table 29-5)
  1. Recurrent bacterial infections reflect the inability of the affected male to produce antibodies.
  2. Treatment is with the intravenous or intramuscular administration of gamma globulin plus antibiotics, when bacterial infection occurs.

Table 29-5. *Disorders of the Immunoglobulins*

X-linked agammaglobulinemia

Acquired hypoimmunoglobulinemia

Selective immunoglobulin A deficiency

Cold autoimmune diseases
  Cryoglobulinemia
  Cold hemagglutinin disease

Multiple myeloma

Waldenström's macroglobulinemia

Amyloidosis

Hyperimmunoglobulinemia E syndrome

Wiskott-Aldrich syndrome

Ataxia-telangiectasia

B. **Selective Immunoglobulin A Deficiency**
   1. Recurrent sinus and pulmonary infections are the most common symptoms, although many patients are asymptomatic; the condition remains undetected until they are screened as potential blood donors.
   2. These patients may develop anti-IgA antibodies and experience a life-threatening anaphylactic reaction, should they be transfused with blood containing IgA.
C. **Cold Autoimmune Diseases** (Table 29-6)
   1. **Cryoglobulinemia** is a disorder in which circulating abnormal proteins (cryoglobulins) precipitate on exposure to cold (usually at a blood temperature <33°C).
   2. **Management of Anesthesia**
      a. An important goal is to maintain body temperature above the thermal reactivity of the cryoglobulin (increase ambient temperature of the operating room, warm and humidify inhaled gases, warm intravenous fluids).
      b. Hypothermic cardiopulmonary bypass and use of cold cardioplegia solutions may not be possible.
D. **Multiple Myeloma**

Table 29-6. *Cold Autoimmune Diseases*

Disease	Thermal Reactivity (°C)	Associated Conditions	Response to Cold Exposure
Cryoglobu-linemia	17–33	Macroglobu-linemia	Hyperviscosity Platelet aggre-gation Renal failure
Cold hemagglu-tinin disease	15–32	None	Acrocyanosis Hemolysis Raynaud's phenomenon
Paroxysmal cold hemoglobinuria	10–15	Syphilis	Hemolysis Jaundice Renal failure
Acquired cold autoimmune disease	4–25	Mycoplasma Mononucleosis Leukemia	Acrocyanosis Hyperviscosity Hemolysis

1. This disease is due to neoplastic proliferation of a single clone of immunoglobulin-secreting cells that invade bone marrow and the skeletal system (Table 29-7).
2. **Treatment** includes chemotherapeutic drugs and corticosteroids, in an effort to decrease the proliferation of plasma cells.
   a. Hypercalcemia may require aggressive treatment (see Chapter 21).
   b. **Plasmapheresis** is usually effective in decreasing viscosity of the blood, as before a blood transfusion to treat anemia.
   c. **Decompression laminectomy** is performed if evidence of spinal cord compression progresses despite treatment.
3. **Management of anesthesia** is influenced by the possible presence of compression fractures and the subsequent impact of positioning during surgery.

E. **Waldenström's Macroglobulinemia**
1. This disease is due to neoplastic proliferation of an IgM-secreting plasma cell that infiltrates bone marrow. It rarely involves the skeletal system (as a result, renal dysfunction due to hypercalcemia is unlikely).
2. **Treatment** is with plasmapheresis to remove the abnormal protein and diminish the viscosity of the plasma.

F. **Amyloidosis**

Table 29-7. *Signs and Symptoms of Multiple Myeloma*

Bone Marrow Invasion
   Thrombocytopenia
   Neutropenia
   Anemia
   Increased susceptibility to infection

Skeletal Invasion
   Pathologic fractures
   Vertebral collapse
   Spinal cord compression (may require urgent laminectomy)
   Hypercalcemia (associated with central nervous system depression and renal dysfunction)

Miscellaneous Findings
   Peripheral neuropathy
   High-output congestive heart failure

1. This disease is characterized by the accumulation of insoluble fibrillar proteins (amyloid) in various tissues (Table 29-8).
2. The frequent presence of amyloid in the rectum makes rectal biopsy an important diagnostic test.
3. Treatment of amyloidosis is generally ineffective.

VIII. DISORDERS OF THE COMPLEMENT SYSTEM

A. Hereditary Angioedema

1. This disease is characterized by uncontrolled activation of the complement pathway (due to absence of C1 esterase inhibitor in the plasma), leading to the release of vasoactive mediators that increase vascular permeability.

   a. As such, hereditary angioedema is characterized by episodic painless edema of the skin (face and limbs) and mucous membranes (respiratory and gastrointestinal tract).

   b. Laryngeal edema is the most dangerous manifestation and can lead to airway obstruction and death.

   c. A typical attack lasts 48 to 72 hours and is most often initiated by trauma, particularly a dental procedure.

2. **Medical Management** (Table 29-9)

3. **Management of Anesthesia**

   a. The most important goal is adequate short-term pro-

Table 29-8. *Sites of Accumulation of Amyloid*

Upper airway (macroglossia contributes to airway obstruction and interferes with direct laryngoscopy)

Salivary glands

Heart (heart block)

Kidneys (nephrotic syndrome)

Gastrointestinal tract (malabsorption, ileus, obstruction)

Peripheral nerves (carpal tunnel syndrome)

Autonomic nervous system (delayed gastric emptying, orthostatic hypotension)

Joints (pain, limited motion)

Table 29-9. *Medical Management of Hereditary Angioedema*

Long-Term Prophylaxis
    Antifibrinolytic agents
        Epsilon aminocaproic acid
        Tranexamic acid
    Anabolic steroids
        Danazol
        Stanazolol

Short-Term Prophylaxis
    Anabolic steroids (2–3 days before surgery)
    Fresh frozen plasma (2 units the day before
      surgery)
    Purified preparation of C1 esterase inhibitor available

Acute Attack
    No specific treatment is reliably effective
    Purified preparation of C1 esterase inhibitor may
      be useful
    Tracheal intubation

Table 29-10. *Examples of Autoimmune Diseases*

Organ-Specific Diseases
    Insulin dependent (type 1) diabetes mellitus
    Myasthenia gravis
    Graves' disease
    Thyroiditis
    Addison's disease
    Pernicious anemia
    Male infertility
    Primary biliary cirrhosis
    Chronic active hepatitis
    Crohn's disease
    Autoimmune hemolytic anemia
    Psoriasis

Systemic Diseases
    Rheumatic fever
    Rheumatoid arthritis
    Ankylosing spondylitis

(Continues)

Table 29-10. *Examples of Autoimmune Diseases* (Continued)

Systemic Diseases *(cont'd)*
Systemic lupus erythematosus
Scleroderma
Polymyositis
Goodpasture syndrome
Chronic graft-versus-host disease
Hypereosinophilic syndrome
Lyme disease
Kawasaki disease
Immunoglobulin A deficiency
Hereditary complement deficiency
Vasculitis
Sarcoidosis

phylaxis before any procedure in which airway trauma, including tracheal intubation, is anticipated.

b. Incidental trauma to the upper airway as produced by an oropharyngeal airway or suctioning should be minimized.

c. Intramuscular injections do not seem to cause any unique problems in these patients.

d. The choice of drugs to produce regional or general anesthesia is not influenced by the presence of hereditary angioedema.

IX. AUTOIMMUNE DISEASE (Table 29-10)

A. Autoimmune disease occurs when the host's own tissues act as self-antigens to evoke the production of autoantibodies.

B. The resulting antigen-antibody interaction produces tissue injury.

CHAPTER 30

Psychiatric Illness and Substance Abuse

The prevalence of psychiatric illness increases the likelihood that such a disorder will be present as a co-existing problem in patients requiring anesthesia (see Stoelting RK, Dierdorf SF. Psychiatric illness and substance abuse. In: Anesthesia and Co-Existing Disease. 3rd Ed. New York. Churchill Livingstone, 1993)).

I. **MENTAL DEPRESSION** is the most common psychiatric disorder (affects 2% to 4% of the adult population) (Table 30-1).

   A. Alcoholism and major depression often occur together.

   B. The risk of suicide is increased in these patients. In the United States, suicide is the 10th leading cause of death and for physicians <40 years of age, it ranks first.

   C. **Treatment** of mental depression is with antidepressant drugs or electroconvulsive therapy (ECT).

   D. **Management of anesthesia** includes continuation of antidepressant drug therapy and consideration of treatment-induced side effects (Tables 30-2 to 30-4).

   1. **Tricyclic antidepressants** may be associated with increased anesthetic requirements, exaggerated responses to vasopressors, tachydysrhythmias in response to administration of pancuronium in the presence of halothane, and the possibility of enhanced seizure activity induced by enflurane. The potential for hypertensive crises is greatest during acute treatment (first 14 to 21 days) with tricyclic antidepressants, whereas chronic treatment is associated with down-regulation of receptors and a decreased likelihood of exaggerated blood pressure responses after administration of a vasopressor.

   2. **Monoamine oxidase inhibitors (MAOIs),** unlike tricyclic antidepressants, have negligible anticholinergic effects and do not produce sedation or sensitize the heart to the dysrhythmogenic effects of epinephrine.

      a. Discontinuation of the MAOI before elective surgery may put the patient at increased risk of suicide. There is a growing appreciation that anesthesia can

Table 30-1. *Characteristics of Major Depression*

Depressed mood

Decreased interest in daily activities and physical appearance

Fluctuations in body weight

Insomnia or hypersomnia

Fatigue

Decreased ability to concentrate

Recurrent thoughts of suicide

Table 30-2. *Tricyclic Antidepressants and Related Antidepressants*

Drugs	Sedative Potency	Anticho-linergic Potency	Orthostatic Hypotension	Cardiac Dysrhythmia Potentiation
Tricyclics				
Doxepin	+++	++	++	++
Amitriptyline	+++	++++	+++	++
Imipramine	++	++	+++	++
Protriptyline	+	+++	+	++
Nortriptyline	+	+	+	++
Desipramine	+	+	+++	++
Related Polycyclics				
Anixaoube	+	+	++	++
Malprotiline	++	+	++	++
Atypical Drugs				
Fluoxetine	+	0	0	+
Trazodone	+++	+	+++	+
Alprazolam	+++	0	0	0

0, none; +, low; ++, moderate; +++, high; ++++, marked.

be safely administered to the patient being treated with a MAOI.

   b. Opioids should probably be avoided in the preoperative medication and in intraoperative management. If opioids are required for postoperative analgesia, morphine and fentanyl are the preferred drugs.

Table 30-3. *Side Effects of Monoamine Oxidase Inhibitor Treatment*

Sedation

Blurred vision

Orthostatic hypotension

Peripheral neuropathy

Hypertension in response to ingestion of tyramine-containing foods

Hyperthermia in response to opioid administration

Table 30-4. *Physiologic Effects of Electroconvulsive Therapy*

Parasympathetic nervous system stimulation
  Bradycardia
  Hypotension
Sympathetic nervous system stimulation
  Tachycardia
  Hypertension
  Cardiac dysrhythmias
Increased cerebral blood flow
Increased intracranial pressure
Increased intraocular pressure
Increased intragastric pressure
Hypoventilation

  c. Epinephrine added to the local anesthetic solution should probably be avoided when a regional anesthetic technique is selected.

  d. Should a vasopressor be required, a direct-acting drug such as phenylephrine is recommended.

3. Electroconvulsive therapy is usually combined with general anesthesia (methohexital 0.5 to 1 mg·kg^{-1} IV) and skeletal muscle paralysis (succinylcholine 0.3 to 0.5 mg·kg^{-1}), to ensure patient comfort and safety.

  a. Administration of an anticholinergic drug intravenously 1 to 2 minutes before induction of anesthesia and delivery of the electrical current may be useful for decreasing the likelihood of bradycardia, which may accompany ECT.

b. Monitoring of the electrocardiogram is useful for recognition of ECT-induced cardiac dysrhythmias.

c. Support of ventilation of the lungs with supplemental oxygen is recommended before the production of the seizure and until the effects of succinylcholine have waned (peripheral nerve stimulator). Apnea lasting up to 2 minutes can follow ECT in the absence of succinylcholine.

d. Monitoring of arterial oxygen saturation with a pulse oximeter is useful in guiding the need for supplemental oxygen and mechanical support of ventilation in the patient undergoing ECT.

II. MANIA is an autosomal dominant disease manifested as a sustained period of mood elevation and in severe cases delusions and hallucinations.

A. Treatment is with lithium and, in severe cases, with an antipsychotic drug (haloperidol).

1. Lithium is absorbed efficiently after oral administration, but its therapeutic (0.6 to 1.2 $mEq \cdot L^{-1}$) to toxic (>2 $mEq \cdot L^{-1}$) ratio is narrow (Table 30-5).

a. A loop or thiazide diuretic that enhances the renal excretion of sodium will increase reabsorption of lithium and increase the plasma concentration by as much as 50%.

b. Administration of sodium-containing solutions and/or an osmotic diuretic will favor the renal excretion of lithium in the patient who manifests evidence of lithium toxicity.

Table 30-5. *Toxic Effects of Lithium*

Skeletal muscle weakness

Ataxia

Sedation

Widening of the QRS complex and heart block

Hypotension

Seizures

2. Carbamazepine is useful in patients who are unresponsive to lithium, recognizing that hepatotoxicity may accompany use of this drug.

B. Management of anesthesia includes evaluation of the presence of lithium toxicity (measure plasma concentration and administer sodium-containing intravenous solutions).

III. SCHIZOPHRENIA is the most common psychotic disorder, accounting for about 20% of all persons treated for mental illness. **Treatment** is with an antipsychotic drug (phenothiazines, butyrophenones) that may be associated with significant side effects including **neuroleptic malignant syndrome** (Table 30-6).

IV. ANXIETY DISORDERS are usually self-limited, although a short course of low-dose benzodiazepine therapy may be instituted (Table 30-7). A **panic disorder** is a discrete period of intense fear (dyspnea, chest pain, fear of dying) that is not triggered by a severe anxiogenic stimulus.

V. AUTISM is a developmental disorder characterized by disturbances in the rate of development of physical, social, and language skills.

VI. SUBSTANCE ABUSE AND DRUG OVERDOSE

Table 30-6. *Side Effects Produced by Antipsychotic Drugs*

Extrapyramidal symptoms
    Acute dystonia (diphenhydramine 25–50 mg IV)
    Tardive dyskinesia

Orthostatic hypotension

Sedation

Neuroleptic malignant syndrome
    Skeletal muscle rigidity
    Hyperthermia (no link with malignant hyperthermia)
    Altered level of consciousness
    Autonomic nervous system instability (tachycardia, labile blood pressure, cardiac dysrhythmias)
    Myoglobinuria and renal failure

Table 30-7. *Manifestations of an Anxiety Disorder*

Tremor

Dyspnea

Tachycardia

Diaphoresis

Insomnia

Irritability

Polyuria

Fatigue

Diarrhea

Skeletal muscle tension

A. **Dependence** is diagnosed on the basis of characteristic symptoms (Table 30-8).
B. Substance abuse is often first suspected or recognized during the medical management of another disorder. Psychiatric consultation is recommended in all cases of substance abuse.
C. **Drug overdose** is the leading cause of unconsciousness observed in patients brought to the emergency department (Table 30-9).

Table 30-8. *Characteristic Symptoms for Psychoactive Drug Dependence*

1. Drug taken in greater dose or for a longer period than intended
2. Unsuccessful attempts to decrease use of drug
3. Increased time spent in obtaining the drug
4. Frequent intoxication or withdrawal symptoms
5. Restricted social or work activities because of drug use
6. Continued drug use despite social or physical problems related to drug use
7. Evidence of tolerance to effects of drug
8. Characteristic withdrawal symptoms
9. Drug use to avoid withdrawal symptoms

Table 30-9. *Evaluation of Depth of Central Nervous System Depression in the Presence of Drug Overdose*

Response to painful stimulation

Activity of gag reflex (absence confirms loss of protective airway reflexes and need for tracheal intubation to protect the lungs from aspiration)

Presence or absence of hypotension

Breathing rate

Size and responsiveness of the pupils

1. The first step in treatment is to secure the airway and support ventilation and circulation.
   a. **Hypothermia** often accompanies unconsciousness due to drug overdose.
   b. A decision to attempt removal of the ingested substance (gastric lavage, forced diuresis, hemodialysis) depends on the drug ingested, the time since ingestion, and the degree of central nervous system depression.
D. **Alcoholism** affects at least 10 million Americans and up to one-third of adult patients have medical problems related to alcohol (Table 30-10).
   1. **Treatment** of alcoholism is total abstinence from alcohol ingestion.

Table 30-10. *Medical Problems Related to Alcoholism*

Central Nervous System Effects
    Psychiatric disorders (depression, antisocial behavior)
    Nutritional disorders (Wernicke-Korsakoff syndrome)
    Withdrawal syndrome
    Cerebellar degeneration
    Cerebral atrophy

Cardiovascular Effects
    Dilated cardiomyopathy
    Cardiac dysrhythmias
    Hypertension

(Continues)

Table 30-10. *Medical Problems Related to Alcoholism* (Continued)

Gastrointestinal and Hepatobiliary Effects
  Esophagitis
  Gastritis
  Pancreatitis
  Hepatic cirrhosis (portal hypertension manifesting as esophageal varices or hemorrhoids)

Skin and Musculoskeletal Effects
  Spider angiomas
  Myopathy
  Osteoporosis

Endocrine and Metabolic Effects
  Decreased plasma testosterone (impotence)
  Decreased gluconeogenesis (hypoglycemia)
  Ketoacidosis
  Hypoalbuminemia
  Hypomagnesemia

Hematologic Effects
  Thrombocytopenia
  Leukopenia
  Anemia

---

2. **Overdose** is treated by maintenance of ventilation (alcohol blood concentration >500 mg·dl^{-1}) and a high index of suspicion of hypoglycemia. **Intoxication** is often defined as a blood alcohol concentration >100 mg·dl^{-1}.
3. **Withdrawal Syndrome** (Table 30-11)
4. **Management of Anesthesia** (see Chapter 18, section IX)

E. **Cocaine**
   1. **Overdose** produces overwhelming sympathetic nervous system stimulation of the cardiovascular system (hypertension, pulmonary edema, coronary artery constriction).
      a. Esmolol or labetalol is useful in blunting the effects of sympathetic nervous system stimulation.
      b. Diazepam may be effective in terminating cocaine-induced seizures.
   2. **Management of anesthesia** in the patient who is acutely intoxicated with cocaine must consider the vulnerabili-

Table 30-11. *Alcohol Withdrawal Syndrome*

Early Manifestations (6–8 hours after decrease in blood alcohol level)
  Generalized tremor
  Autonomic nervous system hyperactivity
  Insomnia
  Agitation

Delirium Tremens (2–4 days after cessation of alcohol ingestion; develops in 5% of patients and is life-threatening)
  Hallucinations
  Combativeness
  Hyperthermia
  Tachycardia
  Hypotension/hypertension
  Seizures

Treatment
  Diazepam (5–10 mg IV every 5 minutes until patient becomes calm)
  Esmolol until heart rate <100 beats·min^{-1}
  Correction of electrolyte (magnesium) and metabolic (thiamine) derangements
  Lidocaine
  Physical restraint

ty of these patients to myocardial ischemia and cardiac dysrhythmias (avoid drugs that stimulate the sympathetic nervous system).

F. Opioids
  1. Dependence rarely develops from use of these drugs to treat acute postoperative pain.
  2. Numerous medical problems, which should be evaluated preoperatively, are likely to be encountered in the opioid addict (Table 30-12).
  3. Overdose (Table 30-13)
  4. Withdrawal syndrome from opioids is unpleasant but is rarely life-threatening (Table 30-14).
  5. Management of Anesthesia (Table 30-15)

G. Barbiturates
  1. Overdose is associated with central nervous system depression, hypoventilation, and hypotension.

Table 30-12. *Medical Problems Associated With Chronic Opioid Abuse*

Cellulitis

Superficial skin abscesses

Septic thrombophlebitis

Tetanus

Endocarditis with or without pulmonary emboli

Systemic septic emboli and infarctions

Aspiration pneumonitis

Acquired immunodeficiency syndrome

Adrenal gland dysfunction

Hepatitis

Malaria

Malnutrition

Positive and false-positive serology

Transverse myelitis

Table 30-13. *Signs and Symptoms of Opioid Overdose*

Slow breathing rate (administer naloxone until >12 breaths•min^{-1})

Normal to increased tidal volume

Miotic pupils

Unconsciousness

Seizures

Pulmonary edema

Arterial hypoxemia

Gastric atony

2. **Withdrawal Syndrome.** In contrast to opioid withdrawal, the abrupt cessation of excessive barbiturate ingestion is associated with potentially life-threatening responses (cardiovascular collapse, seizures) (Table 30-16). Pentobarbital may be administered if signs of barbiturate withdrawal manifest.

3. **Management of anesthesia** is most likely to be influ-

Table 30-14. *Time Course of Opioid Withdrawal Syndrome*

Drug	Onset	Peak Intensity	Duration
Meperidine Dihydromorphine	2–6 h	8–12 h	4–5 d
Codeine Morphine Heroin	6–18 h	36–72 h	7–10 d
Methadone	24–48 h	3–21 d	6–7 wk

Table 30-15. *Management of Anesthesia in the Presence of Opioid Abuse*

Current Opioid Abuse
    Maintain opioid (methadone)
    Volatile anesthetic selected
    Anticipate perioperative hypotension

Rehabilitated Opioid Addict
    Volatile anesthetic selected
    Anticipate exaggerated postoperative pain
      (methadone has minimal analgesic activity)

Table 30-16. *Time Course of Barbiturate Withdrawal Syndrome*

Drug	Onset (h)	Peak Intensity (d)	Duration (d)
Pentobarbital	12–24	2–3	7–10
Secobarbital	12–24	2–3	7–10
Phenobarbital	48–72	6–10	10 days or longer

enced by cross-tolerance with depressant effects of anesthetic drugs.

H. Benzodiazepines, when ingested in excess, produce tolerance and dependence. The combination of benzodiazepines with other depressants (alcohol) may produce exaggerated effects. **Treatment** of an overdose is supportive and administration of a specific benzodiazepine antagonist (**flumazenil**) if depression is profound.

I. **Amphetamines**
   1. **Dependence** is profound. Chronic abuse results in depletion of body stores of catecholamines.
   2. **Overdose** causes anxiety, psychotic states, progressive central nervous system irritability, and cardiovascular stimulation.
   3. **Withdrawal syndrome** is characterized by extreme lethargy and mental depression.
   4. **Management of Anesthesia** (Table 30-17)
J. **Hallucinogens** produce psychological dependence, but there is no evidence of physical dependence or withdrawal symptoms.
   1. **Overdose** is usually not life-threatening. Treatment is symptomatic (calm and quiet environment with minimal external stimuli).
   2. **Management of anesthesia** may be complicated by an acute panic response (treat with diazepam).
K. **Marijuana** abuse is associated with sedation, tachycardia, orthostatic hypotension, and bronchitis, which are considerations in the management of anesthesia in these patients.
L. **Tricyclic antidepressant overdose** is the most common cause of death from drug ingestion (potential lethal dose may only be 5 to 10 times the daily therapeutic dose).
   1. An overdose principally affects the central nervous system, parasympathetic nervous system, and cardiovascular system (Table 30-18).
   2. **Treatment** in the presence of protective upper airway reflexes consists of induced emesis and/or gastric

---

Table 30-17. *Management of Anesthesia in the Presence of Amphetamine Abuse*

Acute Amphetamine Intoxication
    Hypertension
    Tachycardia
    Hyperthermia
    Increased anesthetic requirements
    Exaggerated response to vasopressors

Chronic Amphetamine Intoxication
    Decreased response to vasopressors
    Decreased anesthetic requirements

Table 30-18. *Signs and Symptoms of Tricyclic Antidepressant Drug Overdose*

Seizures

Coma (lasts 24–72 hours)

Intense anticholinergic effects
 Tachycardia
 Mydriasis
 Urinary retention
 Delayed gastric emptying

lavage plus pharmacologic treatment of specific symptoms (Table 30-19).

M. **Salicyclic Acid Overdose** (Table 30-20)

N. **Acetaminophen overdose is** manifested as vomiting, abdominal pain, and life-threatening centrilobular hepatic necrosis (treat with acetylcysteine).

O. **Methyl alcohol ingestion** results in metabolic acidosis, reflecting its metabolism to formaldehyde and formic acid.

 1. A toxic effect of these metabolites on the optic nerve is associated with blindness.

 2. **Treatment** consists of intravenous administration of alcohol, which competes with methyl alcohol for the enzyme alcohol dehydrogenase (same treatment for **ethylene glycol ingestion**).

P. **Petroleum product ingestion** results in hydrocarbon pneumonitis secondary to pulmonary aspiration. Sudden death may reflect a cardiac dysrhythmia.

Table 30-19. *Pharmacologic Treatment of Tricyclic Antidepressant Overdose*

Side Effect	Treatment
Seizures	Diazepam
	Phenytoin
Cardiac dysrhythmias	Lidocaine
	Phenytoin
Heart block	Isoproterenol
Hypotension	Sympathomimetic
	Inotrope

Table 30-20. *Salicylic Acid Overdose*

Symptoms parallel blood salicylate level (>85 mg•dl⁻¹ is severe overdose)

Hyperventilation (resulting alkalosis favors renal excretion of salicylic acid; maintain pH >7.4)

Hypoglycemia

Noncardiogenic pulmonary edema

Hyperthermia

Seizures

Q. Organophosphate overdose leads to excessive accumulation of acetylcholine at nicotinic (neuromuscular junction) and cholinergic receptor sites (Table 30-21). Pharmacologic treatment is necessary to prevent death, which is usually due to apnea (Table 30-22).

R. Carbon monoxide intoxication is the most frequent immediate cause of death from fire-related smoke inhalation (0.1% decreases oxygen carrying capacity of the blood by 50%).

Table 30-21. *Symptoms of Organophosphate (Insecticide) Overdose*

Nicotinic Effects (Neuromuscular Junction)
  Skeletal muscle fasciculations
  Skeletal muscle weakness
  Skeletal muscle paralysis (apnea)

Muscarinic Effects
  Salivation
  Lacrimation
  Miosis
  Diaphoresis
  Bronchospasm
  Bradycardia
  Hyperperistalsis (diarrhea, urination)

Central Nervous System Effects
  Grand mal seizures
  Unconsciousness
  Apnea
  Hyperthermia

Table 30-22. *Treatment of Organophosphate (Insecticide) Overdose*

Drug	Dose
Atropine	2 mg IV until ventilation improves; usual dose for severe toxicity is 15–20 mg during first 3 hours
Pralidoxime	600 mg IV
Diazepam	5–10 mg IV; repeat until seizures are controlled

1. **Diagnosis** is suggested by **measurement of a low SaO_2** in the presence of a normal PaO_2.
   a. Measurement of the blood carboxyhemoglobin concentration confirms the diagnosis (intoxication severe when carboxyhemoglobin concentration >40%).
   b. A high plasma concentration of carboxyhemoglobin can cause the pulse oximeter to overestimate the SaO_2.
   c. Calculation of SaO_2 from a nomogram based on measured PaO_2 will lead to an erroneous conclusion when the plasma carboxyhemoglobin concentration is increased.
2. **Treatment** consists of delivery of maximum inspired concentration of oxygen to speed displacement of carbon monoxide from hemoglobin.

CHAPTER 31

Physiologic Changes and Diseases Unique to the Parturient

Pregnancy and subsequent labor and delivery are accompanied by unique physiologic changes that may be further altered by co-existing disease (see Stoelting RK, Dierdorf SF. Physiologic changes and diseases unique to the parturient. In: Anesthesia and Co-Existing Disease. 3rd Ed. New York. Churchill Livingstone, 1993).

I. PHYSIOLOGIC CHANGES IN PREGNANCY

A. **Cardiovascular system** changes during pregnancy provide for the needs of the developing fetus and prepare the mother for those events that accompany labor and delivery (Table 31-1).

1. **Supine hypotension syndrome** reflects decreased venous return due to obstruction of the inferior vena cava and/or the abdominal aorta by the gravid uterus (most parturients initiate compensatory responses that offset the potential adverse hemodynamic sequelae of this phenomenon).

2. **Aortocaval compression** results in uteroplacental insufficiency and fetal asphyxia due to decreased uterine blood flow (especially if systolic blood pressure is <100 mmHg for >10 to 15 minutes).

3. **Left uterine displacement** is effective in moving the gravid uterus off the inferior vena cava or aorta.

B. **Pulmonary system** changes during pregnancy are manifested as alterations in the upper airway, minute ventilation, lung volumes, and arterial oxygenation (Table 31-2).

C. **Nervous system** changes are characterized by decreased anesthetic requirements such that an alveolar anesthetic concentration that would not produce unconsciousness in a nonpregnant patient may approximate an anesthetizing concentration in a parturient.

D. **Gastrointestinal system** changes make the parturient vulnerable to regurgitation of gastric contents (slowed gastric emptying, increased intragastric pressure, decreased lower

Table 31-1. *Changes in the Cardiovascular System*

	Average Change from Nonpregnant Value (%)
Intravascular fluid volume	+35
Plasma volume	+45
Erythrocyte volume	+20
Cardiac output	+40
Stroke volume	+30
Heart rate	+15
Peripheral circulation	
Systolic blood pressure	No change
Systemic vascular resistance	−15
Diastolic blood pressure	−15
Central venous pressure	No change
Femoral venous pressure	+15

Table 31-2. *Changes in the Pulmonary System*

	Average Change from Nonpregnant Value
Minute ventilation	+50%
Tidal volume	+40%
Breathing rate	+10%
PaO_2	+10 mmHg
$PaCO_2$	−10 mmHg
pHa	No change
Total lung capacity	No change
Vital capacity	No change
Functional residual capacity	−20%
Expiratory reserve volume	−20%
Residual volume	−20%
Airway resistance	−35%
Oxygen consumption	+20%

esophageal sphincter pressure) and to the development of acid pneumonitis, should pulmonary aspiration occur.

1. The increased risk of pulmonary aspiration of gastric contents is the reason for recommending placement of a cuffed tube in the trachea of every parturient to be rendered unconscious with central nervous system depressant drugs.

2. Prophylaxis with drugs to increase gastric fluid pH (oral antacids, histamine H-2 receptor antagonists) or to decrease gastric fluid volume (metoclopramide) may be recommended, although it is difficult to prove the efficacy of this practice.

II. PHYSIOLOGY OF THE UTEROPLACENTAL CIRCULATION

A. The placenta provides for the union of the maternal and fetal circulations (fetal blood arrives through two umbilical arteries, while waste-free blood is delivered to the fetus by a single umbilical vein).

B. The most important determinants of placental function are **uterine blood flow** (directly proportional to blood pressure and inversely proportional to uterine vascular resistance) and the **placental area** available for exchange of nutrients.

C. Unique characteristics of the fetal circulation (75% of the umbilical venous blood passes through the liver; dilution of maternally administered drugs by blood returning from the lower extremities and pelvic viscera of the fetus) protect the fetal brain from exposure to high concentrations of depressant drugs.

III. MATERNAL MEDICATION DURING LABOR
(Table 31-3)

IV. PROGRESS OF LABOR

A. Progress of labor refers to increasing cervical dilation, effacement, and descent of the presenting part with time (Fig. 31-1).

B. **Abnormal Progress of Labor** (Table 31-4)

1. Suggestions that regional anesthesia will prolong the latent phase of labor are difficult to confirm, since the early progress of labor is so variable.

Table 31-3. *Maternal Medication During Labor*

Epidural analgesia

Systemic medications
Benzodiazepines (midazolam 0.5–1 mg IV)
Opioids (meperidine popular, based on the belief that the respiratory center of the newborn is less sensitive to this opioid)
Ketamine (10–15 mg IV when vaginal delivery imminent or regional analgesia incomplete)

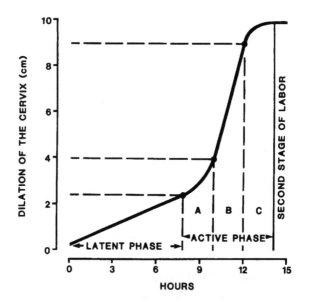

Fig. 31-1. *The progress of labor is described as the first stage (latent and active phase) and second stage, depending on the dilation of the cervix. The active phase consists of the accelerated phase (A), the phase of maximum slope (B), and the deceleration phase (C). (Adapted from Friedman EA. Primigravid labor. A graphicostatistical analysis. Obstet Gynecol 1955;6:567–89, with permission.)*

Table 31-4. *Abnormal Progress of Labor*

	Primigravida	Multigravida	Causes
Slow latent phase	>20 hours	>14 hours	Decreased uterine activity as due to excessive sedation or anesthesia
Active phase arrest	No dilation of cervix for 2 hours	No dilation of cervix for 2 hours	Cephalopelvic disproportion Fetal malposition or malpresentation
Arrest of descent	No descent for 1 hour	No descent for 1 hour	As for active phase arrest

2. During the active phase of labor, a T10 sensory level produced by a regional anesthetic has no significant effect on uterine activity or the progress of labor (provided hypotension is avoided).

3. Regional anesthesia by removing the reflex urge of the parturient to bear down may prolong the second stage of labor.

4. The ability to rapidly achieve an anesthetic concentration of desflurane would be an advantage when rapid uterine relaxation is deemed necessary.

V. REGIONAL ANALGESIA FOR LABOR AND VAGINAL DELIVERY is based on an understanding of the pathways responsible for the transmission of pain during labor and vaginal delivery (Table 31-5 and Fig. 31-2).

VI. INHALATIONAL ANALGESIA FOR VAGINAL DELIVERY as provided by low concentrations of inhaled anesthetic drugs (continuous administration of 30% to 40% nitrous oxide; intermittent inhalation of 0.1% to 0.3% methoxyflurane) is intended to maintain the parturient in an awake and cooperative state with intact laryngeal reflexes.

VII. ANESTHESIA FOR CESAREAN SECTION

A. The choice of anesthetic technique is influenced by both the desires of the patient (regional anesthesia and the

Table 31-5. *Regional Analgesia for Labor and Vaginal Delivery*

Paracervical block (perineal anesthesia only; high incidence of fetal bradycardia)

Lumbar epidural analgesia (segmental band of analgesia preserves pelvic muscle tone; useful during first and second stage of labor)

Caudal analgesia (rarely used)

Spinal anesthesia (increased incidence of postspinal headache)

Pudendal nerve block (administered by the obstetrician just before vaginal delivery)

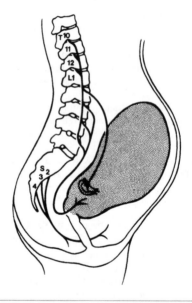

Fig. 31-2. *Schematic diagram of pain pathways during parturition. Afferent pain impulses from the cervix and uterus are carried by nerves that accompany sympathetic nervous system fibers and enter the spinal cord at T10–L1. Pain pathways from the perineum travel to S2–S4 via the pudendal nerves.*

desire to be awake) and urgency of the operation (rapid production of general anesthesia in the presence of fetal distress). Regional anesthesia minimizes the likelihood of maternal pulmonary aspiration and avoids fetal depression.

B. General Anesthesia (Table 31-6)

1. A management plan is useful when a **difficult (failed) intubation** of the parturient's trachea occurs, keeping in mind that the **principal goal is oxygenation without aspiration** (Table 31-7).

2. It is particularly important to minimize the **uterine incision to delivery time.**

C. Regional Anesthesia (Table 31-6)

1. A traditional guide for judging the appropriate dose of local anesthetic to be injected into the subarachnoid space is based on the height of the parturient (Table 31-8).

2. **Postoperative analgesia** may be provided by the inclusion of an opioid in the local anesthetic solution injected into the subarachnoid or epidural space.

Table 31-6. *Anesthesia for Cesarean Section*

General Anesthesia
  Preoperative medication (consider merits of pharmacologic attempts to increase gastric fluid pH; benzodiazepine for anxiety)
  Preoxygenation (vulnerable to arterial hypoxemia with apnea necessary during direct laryngoscopy)
  Induction of anesthesia (thiopental 3–5 mg•kg^{-1} IV plus succinylcholine)
  Maintenance of anesthesia (often only nitrous oxide until delivery of the fetus; after delivery may add a low dose of volatile anesthetic or opioid to reduce the risk of parturient awareness)

Regional Anesthesia
  Spinal anesthesia (technical ease and high success rate; treat systolic blood pressure <100 mmHg with ephedrine 2.5–10 mg IV; a T4–T6 sensory level is necessary)
  Lumbar epidural anesthesia (sensory level more controllable and hypotension less precipitous; limit bupivacaine concentration to 0.5%)

Table 31-7. *Suggested Approach for Management of a Difficult Airway in the Parturient*

Glottic Opening Cannot Be Visualized
    Maintain cricoid pressure
    Summon help
    Repeat direct laryngoscopy
        Optimal head position
        Suction pharynx
        Smaller tracheal tube with stylet
        Temporarily reduce cricoid pressure

If Tracheal Intubation Still Unsuccessful Reapply
Cricoid Pressure and Select the Appropriate Option
    Ventilation Possible—Elective Case
        Maintain cricoid pressure
        Allow patient to awaken
        Select an alternative form of anesthesia
            Regional
            Awake tracheal intubation followed by general anesthesia

    Ventilation Possible—Emergency Case
        Maintain cricoid pressure
        Add an inhalation anesthetic during spontaneous or controlled ventilation
        Expedite delivery and avoid fundal pressure

    Ventilation Impossible
        Maintain cricoid pressure
        Insert an oropharyngeal and/or nasopharyngeal airway
        Summon surgical help
        Cricothyrotomy
        Tracheostomy

(Adapted from Davies JM, Weeks S, Crone LA, Pavlin E. Difficult intubation in the parturient. Can J Anaesth 1989;36:668-74, with permission.)

Table 31-8. *Dose of Local Anesthetic for Spinal Anesthesia Prior to Cesarean Section*

Height (cm)	Tetracaine (mg)	Lidocaine (mg)	Bupivacaine (mg)
<155	7	50	9
155–170	8	60	11
>170	9	70	13

VIII. ABNORMAL PRESENTATIONS AND MULTIPLE BIRTHS

A. Description of fetal position is based on the relationship of the fetal occiput, chin, or sacrum to the left or right side of the parturient (about 90% of deliveries are cephalic presentations in either the occiput transverse or occiput anterior positions).

B. **Persistent occiput posterior** position results in a prolonged and painful labor. A regional anesthetic technique that relaxes the maternal perineal muscles is often avoided until spontaneous internal rotation of the fetal head occurs.

C. **Breech presentation** (feet against the face most common) results in increased maternal morbidity (cervical lacerations, retained placenta, shock due to hemorrhage) and neonatal morbidity and mortality (prolapse of the umbilical cord, intracranial hemorrhage).

   1. **Cesarean delivery** using general or regional anesthesia (remember that uterine hypertonus may require rapid induction of general anesthesia) is often selected for elective delivery of a breech presentation.

   2. **Vaginal delivery** requires that the parturient be able to expel the fetus until the umbilicus is visible. The obstetrician then completes the delivery, either manually or with the application of forceps.

   a. Analgesia during labor is provided with local infiltration, parenteral analgesics, inhalation drugs, or a continuous lumbar epidural technique (0.25% bupivacaine to preserve the ability of the parturient to push).

   b. Rapid induction of general anesthesia may be necessary if perineal muscle relaxation is inadequate for delivery of the aftercoming head or if the lower uterine segment contracts and traps the head.

D. **Multiple gestations** are associated with pregnancy-induced hypertension, prematurity, breech presentation, hemorrhage, and an increased incidence of supine hypotension syndrome (larger uterus produces greater aortocaval compression). Continuous lumbar epidural analgesia is an acceptable technique in these patients.

IX. PREGNANCY AND HEART DISEASE

A. Maternal heart disease is present in about 1.6% of all pregnancies.

1. Many of the signs and symptoms of normal pregnancy (dyspnea, leg edema, flow murmurs) can mimic cardiac disease.
2. Pregnancy and labor often result in circulatory changes (increased cardiac output) that may have adverse effects on the already diseased cardiovascular system.

B. The most common causes of heart disease in the parturient are congenital malformations and acquired valvular heart disease (Table 31-9) (see Chapters 2 and 3).

Table 31-9. *Heart Disease in the Parturient*

Mitral stenosis (most common cardiac valvular defect present during pregnancy; increased incidence of pulmonary edema and atrial tachydysrhythmias; continuous lumbar epidural analgesia useful for labor and vaginal delivery)

Mitral regurgitation (usually tolerate pregnancy well)

Aortic regurgitation (usually tolerate pregnancy well)

Aortic stenosis (vulnerable to decreased stroke volume and hypotension should systemic vascular resistance be abruptly decreased)

Tetralogy of Fallot (pain during labor may increase pulmonary vascular resistance and magnitude of arterial hypoxemia; risk greatest immediately postpartum when systemic vascular resistance is the lowest)

Eisenmenger syndrome (maternal mortality approaches 30%; goal of any anesthetic technique is avoidance of an abrupt decrease in systemic vascular resistance or cardiac output, or an increase in pulmonary vascular resistance)

Coarctation of the aorta (maintenance of heart rate, myocardial contractility, and systemic vascular resistance are important considerations in the management of anesthesia)

Primary pulmonary hypertension (maternal mortality related to congestive heart failure; management of anesthesia includes avoidance of abrupt increases in pulmonary vascular resistance or decreases in systemic vascular resistance)

(Continues)

Table 31-9. *Heart Disease in the Parturient* (Continued)

Cardiomyopathy of pregnancy (avoid abrupt increases in systemic vascular resistance)

Dissecting aneurysm of the aorta (provide a pain-free state and normal to slightly decreased blood pressure)

Prosthetic valve replacement (presence of anticoagulation may influence anesthetic technique)

X. **PREGNANCY-INDUCED HYPERTENSION** (encompasses isolated hypertension, pre-eclampsia, eclampsia) occurs in 5% to 15% of all pregnancies.

   A. **Pathophysiology** (Table 31-10)
   B. **Treatment** (Table 31-11)
   C. **Management of Anesthesia**

Table 31-10. *Manifestations of Pregnancy-Induced Hypertension*

Cerebral edema

Grand mal seizures

Cerebral hemorrhage (accounts for 30–40% of the mortality in these patients)

Hypertension (generalized arteriolar vasoconstriction)

Congestive heart failure

Decreased colloid oncotic pressure

Arterial hypoxemia

Laryngeal edema

Hepatic dysfunction

Oliguric renal failure

Hypovolemia

Disseminated intravascular coagulation

Decreased uterine blood flow

Premature labor and delivery (meconium aspiration common)

Table 31-11. *Treatment of Pregnancy-Induced Hypertension*

Magnesium (decreases irritability of the central nervous system; therapeutic range is 4–6 mEq•L⁻¹; treat toxicity with intravenous calcium)

Antihypertensive drugs
Hydralazine (5–10 mg IV)
Trimethaphan
Nitroprusside (cyanide toxicity a potential consideration)

Digitalis

Mannitol (cerebral edema)

Furosemide (pulmonary edema)

Monitor atrial filling pressures and urine output

Delivery of the fetus and placenta (the definitive therapy)

---

1. A **continuous lumbar epidural technique** is a useful method of analgesia for labor and vaginal delivery in the volume-repleted parturient in good medical control.
   a. Prehydration guided by central venous pressure monitoring is recommended.
   b. Coagulation studies before insertion of the lumbar epidural catheter may be indicated.
   c. Initially, a segmental band of anesthesia (T10–L1) will provide analgesia for uterine contractions. As the second stage of labor is entered, the lumbar epidural anesthetic can be extended, to provide perineal analgesia.
2. **Spinal anesthesia** limited to the sacral area is a consideration when vaginal delivery is imminent.
3. **Cesarean section** is often necessary in the parturient, especially when fetal distress reflects progressive deterioration of the uteroplacental circulation.
   a. General anesthesia (induction with thiopental-succinylcholine) with prehydration and invasive monitoring is often selected. Edema of the upper airway may interfere with visualization of the glottic opening during direct laryngoscopy. Steps to minimize

the pressor response elicited by direct laryngoscopy may be indicated (short-duration laryngoscopy, prior hydralazine or nitroglycerin, introduction of 0.5 MAC volatile anesthetic). Potentiation of muscle relaxants by magnesium therapy is a consideration.

b. Extensive peripheral sympathetic nervous system blockade that may accompany epidural or spinal anesthesia could make management of blood pressure difficult in these patients during cesarean section.

XI. PREGNANCY AND DIABETES MELLITUS (Table 31-12)

XII. MYASTHENIA GRAVIS AND PREGNANCY

A. Anticholinesterase drugs are continued during the pregnancy.

  1. Myasthenia gravis does not affect the course of labor.

  2. A continuous lumbar epidural anesthetic is acceptable for vaginal delivery, recognizing that a high sensory level may have an additive effect with co-existing skeletal muscle weakness.

B. Neonatal myasthenia gravis occurs transiently in 20% to 30% of babies born to mothers with myasthenia gravis.

XIII. HEMORRHAGE IN THE OBSTETRIC PATIENT (Table 31-13)

XIV. ASHERMAN SYNDROME (traumatic intrauterine

Table 31-12. *Pregnancy and Diabetes Mellitus*

Altered insulin requirements (increased in later stages of pregnancy and decreased precipitously during the postpartum period)

Increased risk of ketoacidosis and pregnancy-induced hypertension

Increased neonatal birth weight

Goal is continuation of pregnancy to near term

Elective cesarean section (regional or general anesthesia acceptable)

Table 31-13. *Hemorrhage in the Obstetric Patient*

	Clinical Features	Predisposing Conditions
Placenta previa	Painless vaginal bleeding	Advanced age Multiple parity
Abruptio placentae	Abdominal pain Bleeding partially or wholly concealed Uterine irritability Shock Coagulopathy Acute renal failure Fetal distress	Multiple parity Uterine anomalies Compression of the inferior vena cava Chronic hypertension
Uterine rupture	Severe abdominal pain Shock Disappearance of fetal heart tones	Previous uterine incision Rapid spontaneous delivery Excessive uterine stimulation Cephalopelvic disproportion Multiple parity Polyhydramnios Spontaneous
Retained placenta	Requires uterine relaxation and manual removal of the placenta	
Uterine atony	Complete atony may result in 2000-ml blood loss in 5 minutes Treatment is intravenous oxytocin	Multiple parity Polyhydramnios Large fetus Retained placenta

synechiae) is associated with antepartum and postpartum hemorrhage caused by accretion of the placenta. Emergency hysterectomy may be necessary.

XV. AMNIOTIC FLUID EMBOLISM is signaled by the sudden onset of respiratory distress, profound hypotension, and arterial hypoxemia, often in association with a tumultuous labor.

A. Treatment is symptomatic, and mortality is more than 80%.

B. Conditions that mimic amniotic fluid embolism include inhalation of gastric contents (bronchospasm likely), pulmonary embolism, air embolism, and local anesthetic toxicity.

XVI. ANESTHESIA FOR OPERATIONS DURING PREGNANCY (Table 31-14)

XVII. DIAGNOSIS AND MANAGEMENT OF FETAL DISTRESS is most often based on **electronic fetal monitoring.** This technique permits evaluation of fetal well-being by following fetal changes in heart rate, as recorded using an external monitor (Doppler) or fetal scalp electrode (Figs. 31-3 to 31-5).

XVIII. EVALUATION OF THE FETUS may include amniotic fluid analysis (fetal lung maturity) and ultrasonography (fetal biparietal diameter parallels fetal age; detects fetal defects).

XIX. EVALUATION OF THE NEONATE is designed for

Table 31-14. *Anesthesia for Operations During Pregnancy*

Avoid teratogenic drugs (critical period of organogenesis is 15–56 days of gestation; nitrous oxide is a controversial selection)

Avoid intrauterine fetal hypoxia and acidosis (avoid maternal hypotension, arterial hypoxemia, and excessive changes in $PaCO_2$)

Prevent premature labor (beta-2 agonists may be associated with pulmonary edema, cardiac dysrhythmias, and hypokalemia)

Defer elective surgery until after delivery

Emergency surgery (regional or general anesthesia acceptable; nitrous oxide is a controversial selection; fetal heart rate monitoring; supplemental oxygen)

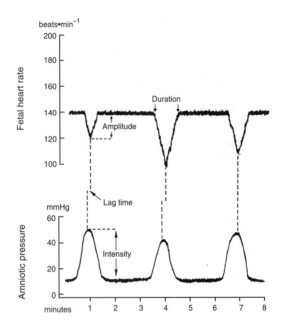

Fig. 31-3. *Early decelerations of the fetal heart rate are characterized by a short lag time between the onset of uterine contractions and the beginning of fetal heart rate slowing. Maximum heart rate slowing is usually <20 beats•min^{-1} and occurs at the peak intensity of the contraction. Heart rate returns to normal by the time the contraction has ceased. The most likely explanation for this early deceleration is a vagal reflex response to compression of the fetal head. (From Shnider SM. Diagnosis of fetal distress: Fetal heart rate. In: Shnider SM, ed. Obstetrical Anesthesia: Current Concepts and Practice. Baltimore. Williams & Wilkins 1970:197–203, with permission.)*

prompt identification of the depressed infant requiring active resuscitation. As a guide to identifying and treating the depressed neonate, the Apgar score has not been surpassed (Table 31-15).

XX. IMMEDIATE NEONATAL PERIOD (Table 31-16) (see Chapter 32)
XXI. POSTPARTUM TUBAL LIGATION is the most

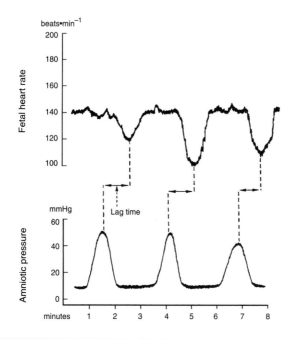

Fig. 31-4. *Late decelerations of the fetal heart rate are characterized by a delay (lag time) between the onset of the uterine contraction and the beginning of fetal heart rate slowing. The fetal heart rate does not return to normal until after the contraction has ceased. A mild late deceleration pattern is present when slowing is <20 beats•min⁻¹. Profound slowing is present when fetal heart rate slows >40 beats•min⁻¹. Late fetal heart rate decelerations indicate fetal distress, owing to uteroplacental insufficiency. (From Shnider SM. Diagnosis of fetal distress: Fetal heart rate. In: Shnider SM, ed. Obstetrical Anesthesia: Current Concepts and Practice. Baltimore. Williams & Wilkins 1970:197–203, with permission.)*

common type of surgery performed during the early post-partum period.

A. Residual anesthesia from delivery may be used, recognizing that a T5 sensory level is necessary to ensure patient comfort.

B. If surgery is delayed 8 to 12 hours postpartum, either general anesthesia or regional anesthesia may be selected.

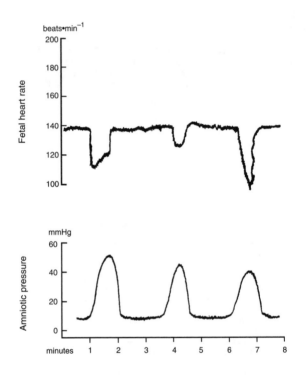

Fig. 31-5. *Variable decelerations of the fetal heart rate are characterized by decreases in the heart rate of varying magnitude and duration that do not show a consistent relationship to uterine contractions. This pattern of fetal heart rate slowing is associated with umbilical cord compression. (From Shnider SM. Diagnosis of fetal distress: Fetal heart rate. In: Shnider SM, ed. Obstetrical Anesthesia: Current Concepts and Practice. Baltimore. Williams & Wilkins 1970:197–203, with permission.)*

Table 31-15. *Evaluation of the Neonate Using the Apgar Score*

Factor	0	1	2
Heart rate (beats·min⁻¹)	Absent	<100	>100
Respiratory effort	Absent	Slow Irregular	Crying
Reflex irritability	No response	Grimace	Crying
Muscle tone	Limp	Flexion of extremities	Active
Color	Pale Cyanotic	Body pink Extremities cyanotic	Pink

Table 31-16. *Abnormalities Present at Birth or Manifested Shortly After Delivery*

Meconium aspiration

Choanal stenosis and atresia

Diaphragmatic hernia

Hypovolemia

Hypoglycemia

Tracheoesophageal fistula

Laryngeal anomalies

Pierre Robin syndrome

CHAPTER 32

Diseases Common to the Pediatric Patient

The pediatric patient (especially the neonate, defined as 0 to 28 days of age) presents unique anatomic, physiologic, and pharmacologic considerations in the management of anesthesia in the presence of diseases that occur exclusively or with an increased frequency in this age group (see Stoelting RK, Dierdorf SF. Diseases common to the pediatric patient. In: Anesthesia and Co-Existing Disease. 3rd Ed. New York. Churchill Livingstone, 1993).

I. ANATOMY OF THE AIRWAY (Table 32-1)

II. PHYSIOLOGY

A. **Respiratory System.** The single most important difference that physiologically distinguishes the pediatric patient from the adult patient is oxygen consumption (Table 32-2).

B. **Cardiovascular System.** The neonate is highly dependent on heart rate for maintenance of cardiac output and blood pressure.

C. **Distribution of Body Water**
   1. Until 18 to 24 months of age, the child's extracellular fluid volume is equivalent to about 40% of body weight, compared with about 20% in an adult.
   2. Intraoperative fluid replacement may be considered as maintenance fluid (often a glucose-containing solution) and replacement fluid (Table 32-3).

D. **Hematology** (Table 32-4)
   1. Acceptable intraoperative blood loss guidelines are based on an **estimated blood volume of 85 ml·kg^{-1}.**
   2. The need for routine preoperative hemoglobin determinations in patients >1 year of age is controversial.

E. **Thermoregulation.** The neonate and infant are vulnerable to hypothermia during the perioperative period. It is crucial to increase the ambient temperature of the operating room.

III. PHARMACOLOGY AND PHARMACOKINETICS

A. **Anesthetic Requirements** (Fig. 32-1)

B. **Muscle Relaxants**

Table 32-1. *Endotracheal Tube Size*

Weight or Age	Internal Diameter[a] (mm)	Distance of Tube Insertion for Midtracheal Position (cm)
1 kg	2.5 uncuffed	7
1.5 kg	3.0 uncuffed	7.5
2 kg	3.0 uncuffed	8
3 kg (preterm)	3.0 uncuffed	9
3 kg (term)	3.0 uncuffed	10
6–12 mo	3.5 uncuffed	11
12–18 mo	3.5 uncuffed	12
18–36 mo	4.0 uncuffed	13
3–5 y	4.5 uncuffed	14
5–6 y	5.0 cuffed	15
6–8 y	5.5 cuffed	16
8–10 y	6.0 cuffed	18
10–12 y	6.5 cuffed	18

[a]Endotracheal tube size for an uncuffed tube should result in an audible air leak when positive airway pressure equivalent to 25 cm H_2O is applied.

Table 32-2. *Mean Pulmonary Function Values*

	Neonate (3 kg)	Adult (70 kg)
Oxygen consumption ($ml \cdot kg^{-1} \cdot min^{-1}$)	6.4	3.5
Alveolar ventilation ($ml \cdot kg^{-1} \cdot min^{-1}$)	130	60
Carbon dioxide production ($ml \cdot kg^{-1} \cdot min^{-1}$)	6	3
Tidal volume ($ml \cdot kg^{-1}$)	6	6
Breathing frequency (min)	35	15
Vital capacity ($ml \cdot kg^{-1}$)	35	70
Functional residual capacity ($ml \cdot kg^{-1}$)	30	35
Tracheal length (cm)	5.5	12
PaO_2 (F_IO_2 0.21, mmHg)	65–85	85–95
$PaCO_2$ (mmHg)	30–36	36–44
pH	7.34–7.40	7.36–7.44

Table 32-3. *Intraoperative Fluid Therapy for the Pediatric Patient*

| Surgical Procedure | 5% Dextrose in Lactated Ringer's Solution (ml·kg^{-1}·h^{-1}) | | |
	Maintenance	Replacement	Total
Minor surgery (herniorrhaphy)	4	2	6
Moderate surgery (pyloromyotomy)	4	4	8
Extensive surgery (bowel resection)	4	6	10

Table 32-4. *Normal Hemogram Values*

Age	Hemoglobin (g·dl^{-1})	Hematocrit (%)	Leukocytes (cells·mm^{-3})
1 d	19.0	61	18,000
2 wk	17.3	54	12,000
1 mo	14.2	43	
2 mo	10.7	31	
6 mo	12.3	36	10,000
1 y	11.6	35	
6 y	12.7	38	
10–12 y	13.0	39	8000

1. Infants are more sensitive to the effects of nondepolarizing muscle relaxants. Because of the relatively large volume of distribution, however, the initial dose of a nondepolarizing muscle relaxant calculated on the basis of the infant's body weight is not different from that of an adult.

2. The neonate and infant require more succinylcholine (2 mg·kg^{-1} IV) than do older children (1 mg·kg^{-1} IV) to produce equivalent degrees of neuromuscular blockade.

3. Diminished hepatic and renal clearance of drugs char-

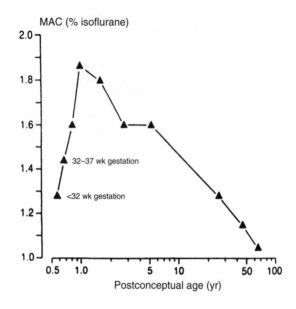

Fig. 32-1. *Anesthetic requirements (MAC) of isoflurane and postconceptual age. (From LeDez KM, Lerman J. The minimum alveolar concentration (MAC) of isoflurane in preterm neonates. Anesthesiology 1987;67:301–7, with permission.)*

acteristic of the neonate can produce prolonged drug effects.

IV. MONITORING DURING THE PERIOPERATIVE PERIOD (Table 32-5)

V. NEONATAL MEDICAL DISEASES (Table 32-6)

VI. NEONATAL SURGICAL DISEASES

A. **Diaphragmatic hernia** results from incomplete embryologic closure of the diaphragm, with subsequent herniation of abdominal contents into the thorax and interference with normal fetal lung maturation (varying degrees of pulmonary hypoplasia).

Table 32-5. *Monitoring of the Pediatric Patient During the Perioperative Period*

Electrocardiogram (cardiac rhythm rather than myocardial ischemia)

Blood pressure (noninvasive vs. intra-arterial catheter; right radial artery a preductal site)

Body temperature

Precordial or esophageal stethoscope

Pulse oximeter

Capnography (limited by small tidal volume or presence of leak around the tracheal tube)

Table 32-6. *Neonatal Medical Diseases*

Respiratory distress syndrome (alveolar collapse results in right-to-left intrapulmonary shunting and arterial hypoxemia; pneumothorax a danger of mechanical ventilation)

Bronchopulmonary dysplasia (chronic phase of respiratory distress syndrome characterized by airway hyperreactivity and arterial hypoxemia)

Intracranial hemorrhage (prematurity the greatest risk factor)

Retinopathy of prematurity (risk neglibible after 44 weeks postconception; maintain PaO_2 60–80 mmHg in a susceptible infant; use nitrous oxide or air to dilute the delivered concentration of oxygen)

Apnea spells (risk decreased beyond 60 weeks postconception; limits outpatient surgery)

Sudden infant death syndrome

Kernicterus

Hypoglycemia

Hypocalcemia (citrate-induced during blood transfusion)

Sepsis (presentation in infant often nonspecific; lethargy, ventilatory distress)

1. **Signs and Symptoms** (Table 32-7)
2. **Treatment** includes prompt decompression of the stomach and administration of supplemental oxygen (often through a tracheal tube).
3. **Management of Anesthesia** (Table 32-8)
4. **Postoperative Management**
    a. After surgical reduction of the hernia, oxygenation may rapidly improve, followed by sudden deterioration with profound arterial hypoxemia (reappearance of fetal circulation pattern).
    b. Prognosis is ultimately determined by the degree of pulmonary hypoplasia. There is no effective treatment for pulmonary hypoplasia, other than keeping the infant alive with the hope that lung maturation will occur (**extracorporeal membrane oxygenation**).

Table 32-7. *Signs and Symptoms of Diaphragmatic Hernia*

Scaphoid abdomen

Barrel-shaped chest

Abdominal contents present in thorax (auscultation, radiograph)

Arterial hypoxemia

Increased pulmonary vascular resistance

Congenital heart disease

Table 32-8. *Management of Anesthesia for Treatment of Diaphagmatic Hernia*

Awake intubation of the trachea

Invasive monitoring of blood pressure (consider preductal artery)

Volatile anesthetic versus opioid with muscle relaxant (avoid nitrous oxide)

Mechanical ventilation of lungs (maintain airway pressure <30 cm H_2O, to minimize risk of pneumothorax)

Attempts to inflate the hypoplastic lung not recommended

B. **Tracheoesophageal fistula** is most often characterized as a blind upper esophageal pouch plus a fistula between the lower esophagus and trachea.
   1. **Signs and Symptoms** (Table 32-9)
   2. **Treatment** is an initial gastrostomy, followed by stabilization and definitive repair of the lesion in 48 to 72 hours.
   3. **Management of Anesthesia** (Table 32-10)
C. **Abdominal Wall Defects** (Table 32-11)
   1. **Preoperative preparation** is based on prevention of infection and minimization of fluid and heat loss from exposed abdominal viscera.
   2. **Management of Anesthesia** (Table 32-12)
D. **Pyloric Stenosis**
   1. **Signs and symptoms** of pyloric stenosis are characterized by persistent vomiting and loss of hydrogen ions, leading to hypovolemia and the development of hypokalemic hypochloremic metabolic alkalosis.

Table 32-9. *Signs and Symptoms of Tracheoesophageal Fistula*

Inability to pass an oral catheter into the stomach

Cyanosis and coughing during oral feeding

Pulmonary aspiration

Gastric distension

Congenital heart disease

Prematurity

Table 32-10. *Management of Anesthesia for Correction of Tracheoesophageal Fistula*

Position tracheal tube below the tracheoesophageal fistula

Volatile anesthetic if adequately hydrated (nitrous oxide or air to dilute delivered oxygen concentration)

Intra-arterial monitoring

Tracheal collapse after extubation may reflect decreased supporting cartilage

Table 32-11. *Abdominal Wall Defects*

Omphalocele	Gastroschisis
External herniation of abdominal viscera through the base of the umbilical cord (hernia sac intact)	External herniation of abdominal viscera through a defect in the abdominal wall (absent hernia sac)
Congenital heart disease likely	Associated congenital anomalies unlikely
Prematurity possible	Prematurity likely

Table 32-12. *Management of Anesthesia for Repair of Abdominal Wall Defects*

Awake intubation of the trachea after gastric decompression

Continue fluid resuscitation

Maintain body temperature

Volatile anesthetic versus opioids (nitrous oxide could contribute to bowel distension)

Muscle relaxants versus feasibility of primary abdominal surgical closure (monitor airway pressure)

Postoperative ventilation of the lungs likely

2. **Treatment** consists of intravenous fluid and electrolyte replacement followed in 24 to 48 hours by elective surgical correction.
3. **Management of Anesthesia** (Table 32-13)
4. **Postoperative management** is influenced by the occasional unexpected occurrence of hypoventilation and hypoglycemia.
E. **Lobar emphysema** is a rare cause of respiratory distress, reflecting compression of normal lung and interference with venous return produced by the overdistended lobe. **Management of anesthesia** is influenced by the possible detrimental effects of positive-pressure ventilation of the lungs (maintain spontaneous ventilation until the chest is open) and nitrous oxide (cause further distension of the diseased lobe).

Table 32-13. *Management of Anesthesia for Treatment of Pyloric Stenosis*

Awake tracheal intubation versus rapid sequence induction (consider risks of pulmonary aspiration and strength of infant)

Volatile anesthetic with or without nitrous oxide

Skeletal muscle relaxants not needed routinely

Mechanical ventilation of the lungs

F. Necrotizing enterocolitis is primarily a disease of preterm neonates that manifests as hypovolemic shock, metabolic acidosis, thrombocytopenia, and peritonitis secondary to multiple bowel preparations. Surgery is reserved for those neonates in whom medical treatment has failed (Table 32-14).

VII. TRAUMA is the leading cause of death in children >1 year of age (blunt head injury) (Table 32-15).

VIII. NERVOUS SYSTEM (Table 32-16)

IX. CRANIOFACIAL ABNORMALITIES

A. Cleft lip and palate are often associated with other congenital anomalies (heart disease), pulmonary aspiration, upper respiratory tract infections, and anemia.

    1. Treatment of cleft lip is cheiloplasty at 2 to 3 months of

Table 32-14. *Management of Anesthesia for Treatment of Necrotizing Enterocolitis*

Monitor adequacy of fluid resuscitation and coagulation

Invasive monitoring of blood pressure

Ketamine and/or opioids plus a muscle relaxant (volatile anesthetics may produce hypotension especially if hypovolemia present)

Avoid nitrous oxide (gas bubbles in mesenteric veins and portal venous system)

Postoperative mechanical ventilation of lungs

Table 32-15. *Preventable Causes of Death Caused by Pediatric Trauma*

Airway obstruction

Pneumothorax

Intra-abdominal bleeding

Expanding intracranial hematoma (Glasgow Coma Scale; see Table 17-13)

Table 32-16. *Diseases of the Nervous System That Afflict Pediatric Patients*

Cerebral palsy (skeletal muscle spasticity and seizures; at risk of pulmonary aspiration; succinylcholine acceptable)

Hydrocephalus (obstructive or nonobstructive; possibility of increased intracranial pressure; air embolism a risk during shunt insertion)

Myelomeningocele (succinylcholine acceptable; increased incidence of latex allergy)

Craniostenosis (possibility of increased intracranial pressure; blood loss likely with corrective surgery)

Epilepsy (see Chapter 17)

Trisomy-21 (atlantoaxial instability and congenital heart disease are considerations)

Neurofibromatosis (see Chapter 17)

Reye syndrome (increased intracranial pressure, coagulopathy, and liver failure)

age. Treatment of cleft palate is palatoplasty at about 18 months of age.

    2. Management of Anesthesia (Table 32-17)

B. Mandibular hypoplasia is a prominent feature of **Pierre Robin, Treacher Collins** (cleft palate and congenital heart disease common), and **Goldenhar syndromes. Management of anesthesia** is influenced by the predictable upper airway obstruction and difficult tracheal intubation (awake versus spontaneous breathing, avoid muscle relaxants) associated with these syndromes. Use of a laryngeal mask airway may be a consideration in these patients.

Table 32-17. *Management of Anesthesia for Surgical Treatment of Cleft Lip and Cleft Palate*

Induction technique (intravenous with muscle relaxant versus maintenance of spontaneous ventilation; influenced by degree of airway abnormality)

Tape tracheal tube to lower lip in midline

Drugs selected for maintenance may be influenced by associated congenital diseases and surgeon's decision to infiltrate the operative site with epinephrine)

Capnography (early warning of tracheal tube displacement)

Protect eyes

Postoperative airway obstruction (especially after palatoplasty)

C. **Hypertelorism** (increased distance between the eyes, as well as other craniofacial anomalies) may be treated surgically (long, complex operations). **Management of anesthesia** presents many potential problems (Table 32-18).

X. DISORDERS OF THE UPPER AIRWAY

A. Epiglottitis (supraglottitis) is a short-lived disease that usually presents with characteristic signs and symptoms (Table 32-19).

1. **Treatment** includes antibiotics (ampicillin) and a

Table 32-18. *Anesthetic Considerations in Management of Craniofacial Surgery*

Difficult tracheal intubation versus elective tracheostomy

Excessive blood loss

Hypothermia

Intracranial hypertension

Corneal abrasions

Invasive monitoring

Postoperative mechanical ventilation of the lungs

secured airway (translaryngeal intubation during general anesthesia is recommended).

   a. An attempt to visualize the epiglottis should not be undertaken until the child is in the operating room and preparations are completed for intubation of the trachea and possible emergency tracheostomy (Table 32-20).

   b. Total upper airway obstruction can occur at any time.

B. **Laryngotracheobronchitis** (croup) is a viral infection of the upper respiratory tract that usually presents with characteristic signs and symptoms (Table 32-19).

   1. **Treatment** includes supplemental oxygen, humidification of inspired gases, and aerosolized racemic epinephrine. Corticosteroids remain controversial therapy.

   2. Tracheal intubation is required if physical exhaustion occurs as evidenced by an increased $PaCO_2$.

Table 32-19. *Clinical Features of Epiglottitis (Supraglottitis) and Laryngotracheobronchitis*

	Epiglottitis	**Laryngotracheobronchitis**
Age group affected	2–6 years	≤2 years
Incidence	Accounts for 5% of children with stridor	Accounts for about 80% of children with stridor
Etiologic agent	Bacterial (*Haemophilus influenzae*)	Viral
Onset	Rapid over 24 hours	Gradual over 24–72 hours
Signs and symptoms	Inspiratory stridor Pharyngitis Drooling Fever (often >39°C) Lethargic to restless Insists on sitting up and leaning forward Tachypnea Cyanosis	Inspiratory stridor Croupy cough Rhinorrhea Fever (rarely >39°C)

(Continues)

Table 32-19. *Clinical Features of Epiglottitis (Supraglottitis) and Laryngotracheobronchitis* (Continued)

	Epiglottitis	Laryngotracheo-obronchitis
Laboratory	Neutrophilia	Lymphocytosis
Lateral radiograph of the neck	Swollen epiglottis	Narrowing of the subglottic area
Treatment	Oxygen	Oxygen
	Urgent intubation of the trachea or tracheostomy during general anesthesia	Aerosolized racemic eprinepherine
		Humidity
	Fluids	Fluids
	Antibiotics	Corticosteroids
	Corticosteroids(?)	Intubation of the trachea for severe airway obstruction

Table 32-20. *Management of Anesthesia in the Treatment of Epiglottitis*

Place an intravenous catheter (consider administration of an anticholinergic drug)

Preparation for emergency cricothyrotomy or tracheostomy

Induction with a volatile anesthetic (halothane)

Direct laryngoscopy for tracheal intubation (and confirmation of diagnosis) when adequate depth of anesthesia achieved

Replace orotracheal tube with a nasotracheal intubation

Consider tracheal extubation (in the operating room) when evidence that edema has subsided (air leak around tracheal tube)

  C. Postintubation laryngeal edema is greatest in children between the ages of 1 and 4 years.
    1. Predisposing factors include mechanical trauma to the airway during placement of the tube, co-existing upper respiratory tract infection, and placement of a tube that

produces a tight fit (recommend air leak during positive airway pressures equivalent to 15 to 25 cm H_2O).

2. **Treatment** is with humidification of inspired gases and aerosolized racemic epinephrine (0.05 ml·kg^{-1} in 2 ml saline) administered hourly until symptoms subside.

   a. **Efficacy of corticosteroids is not documented.**

   b. **Reintubation of the trachea is required rarely.**

D. **Foreign body aspiration** is most likely in children aged 1 to 3 years.

1. **Signs and symptoms** include cough, wheezing, and decreased air entry into the affected lung (may mimic upper respiratory tract infection, asthma, or pneumonia). If the aspirated object is radiolucent, indirect evidence can be obtained by demonstrating hyperinflation of the affected lung with atelectasis distal to the foreign body.

2. **Treatment** consists of endoscopic removal of the foreign body within 24 hours of aspiration.

3. **Management of anesthesia** is influenced by the severity of airway obstruction (topical anesthesia applied after adequate depth of anesthesia achieved, spontaneous ventilation maintained with a volatile anesthetic in oxygen).

   a. Skeletal muscle paralysis may be required for removal of the bronchoscope and foreign body if the object is too large to pass through the moving vocal cords.

   b. Subglottic edema after bronchoscopy may be treated with aerosolized racemic epinephrine and intravenous administration of dexamethasone.

   c. A chest radiograph should be obtained after bronchoscopy for detection of atelectasis or pneumothorax.

E. **Laryngeal papillomatosis** may require surgical therapy with laser coagulation (necessitates skeletal muscle paralysis to produce quiescent vocal cords and precautions against airway fires).

F. **Lung abscess** may require surgical drainage using an anesthetic technique that incorporates a double-lumen tracheal tube or bronchial blocker.

XI. **JEUNE SYNDROME** is an inherited disorder characterized by deformity of the chest wall leading to ventilatory failure (asphyxiating thoracic dystrophy).

XII. MALIGNANT HYPERTHERMIA

  A. Signs and Symptoms (Table 32-21)

  B. Treatment is divided into **etiologic** and **symptomatic** (Table 32-22).

  C. Identification of Susceptible Patients

    1. Prior anesthetic history is important, although a negative history does not always indicate that a patient is not susceptible.

    2. Myopathic syndromes may be associated with an increased risk of malignant hyperthermia.

Table 32-21. *Signs and Symptoms of Malignant Hyperthermia*

Increased carbon dioxide production ($PaCO_2$ >100 mmHg; pH <7.15)

Tachycardia (early sign)

Cardiac dysrhythmias

Arterial hypoxemia

Increased body temperature (may be a late sign)

Masseter muscle spasm after administration of succinylcholine (an estimated 50% of such patients are susceptible to malignant hyperthermia)

Increased plasma creatine kinase and myoglobin concentrations

---

Table 32-22. *Treatment of Malignant Hyperthermia*

Etiologic Treatment
    Dantrolene (2–3 mg•kg^{-1} IV) as an initial bolus, followed with repeat doses every 5–10 minutes until symptoms are controlled (rarely need total dose >10 mg•kg^{-1})
    Prevent recrudescence (dantrolene 1 mg•kg^{-1} IV every 6 hours for 72 hours)

Symptomatic Treatment
    Immediately terminate inhaled anesthetics and conclude surgery as soon as possible
    Hyperventilate the lungs with 100% oxygen

(Continues)

Table 32-22. *Treatment of Malignant Hyperthermia* (Continued)

> Symptomatic Treatment *(cont'd)*
>   Initiate active cooling (iced saline 15 ml•kg^{-1} IV
>   every 10 minutes, gastric lavage with iced saline,
>   surface cooling)
>   Correct metabolic acidosis (sodium bicarbonate
>   1–2 mEq•kg^{-1} IV based on arterial pH)
>   Maintain urine output (hydration, mannitol 0.25
>   g•kg^{-1} IV, furosemide 1 mg•kg^{-1} IV)
>   Treat cardiac dysrhythmias (procainamide 15
>   mg•kg^{-1} IV)
>   Monitor in an intensive care unit (urine output,
>   arterial blood gases, pH, electrolytes)

3. About 70% of susceptible patients have elevations of resting plasma concentrations of creatine kinase.
4. **Skeletal muscle biopsy** (vastus muscle of the thigh) subjected to in vitro isometric contracture testing (caffeine and/or halothane) is the definitive test for confirming susceptibility to malignant hyperthermia.

D. **Management of Anesthesia**
   1. **Prophylaxis** is provided with oral administration of dantrolene 5 mg•kg^{-1} in three or four divided doses every 6 hours, with the last dose given 4 hours preoperatively.
      a. An alternative to oral prophylaxis is administration of dantrolene 2.4 mg•kg^{-1} IV just prior to induction of anesthesia, followed by 1.2 mg•kg^{-1} IV in 6 hours.
      b. Large doses of dantrolene administered as prophylaxis may cause skeletal muscle weakness of sufficient magnitude to interfere with adequate ventilation or protection of the lungs from aspiration of gastric fluid. For this reason, prophylactic use of dantrolene may not be necessary, if all known triggering drugs are avoided (Table 32-23).
   2. **Induction and maintenance** of anesthesia should be restricted to use of nontriggering drugs (Table 32-23).
   3. The anesthesia machine is prepared by a continuous flow of oxygen (10 L•min^{-1}) for 5 minutes and the use of a disposable anesthetic circuit.
   4. Regional anesthesia is acceptable but does not protect against stress-induced malignant hyperthermia.

Table 32-23. *Nontriggering Drugs for Malignant Hyperthermia*

> Barbiturates
> Opioids
> Benzodiazepines
> Propofol
> Etomidate
> Droperidol
> Nitrous oxide
> Nondepolarizing muscle relaxants (*d*-tubocurarine?)
> Anticholinesterases
> Anticholinergics
> Sympathomimetics
> Local anesthetics

XIII. FAMILIAL DYSAUTONOMIA is characterized by dysfunction of the autonomic nervous system (lability of blood pressure, decreased pain perception, vomiting crises with pulmonary aspiration and dehydration, hyperthermia) and development of kyphoscoliosis.

XIV. SOLID TUMORS (Table 32-24)

XV. THERMAL (BURN) INJURY and subsequent survival depends on the age of the patient and the percentage of body area burned.

  A. Pathophysiology. Thermal injury produces predictable pathophysiologic responses (Table 32-25).

  B. Management of anesthesia is influenced by the pathophysiologic responses that accompany thermal injury (Table 32-25).

  1. Sites for intravenous access or placement of monitors may be limited.

  2. Preoperative evaluation of blood glucose concentration (total parenteral nutrition), coagulation status (split-thickness skin graft associated with about 80 ml blood loss for each 100 cm^2 skin harvested), and adequacy of intravascular fluid resuscitation (urine output) may be indicated.

Table 32-24. *Solid Tumors in Children*

Leukemia involving liver and spleen

Hydronephrosis

Neuroblastoma (malignant proliferation of sympathetic ganglion cell precursors)

Nephroblastoma (Wilms tumor) (surgical treatment may predispose to sudden and excessive blood loss)

Table 32-25. *Pathophysiologic Responses Evoked by Burn Injury*

Initial decrease in cardiac output, followed by a hyperdynamic circulation

Hypovolemia (treat within first 24 hours with crystalloids 4 ml•kg^{-1} IV for each percentage of body surface area burn; after 24 hours decrease infusion rate and use colloids, as capillary integrity now improved)

Hypertension

Upper airway edema (hoarseness an indication for tracheal intubation)

Chemical pneumonitis

Carbon monoxide poisoning (see Chapter 30)

Increased metabolic rate

Adynamic ileus

Gastric or duodenal ulcer

Oliguria

Initial hyperkalemia, followed by hypokalemia

Hyperglycemia

Hyperviscosity of blood

Hypercoagulable state

Depression of immune function

3. Measures designed to decrease intraoperative heat loss (radiant warmers, warmed intravenous fluids, increased ambient temperature) are indicated.
4. **Altered Drug Responses** (Table 32-26)

Table 32-26. *Altered Drug Responses in the Thermal Injury Patient*

Thiopental requirements increased

Opioid requirements may be increased

Succinylcholine-induced hyperkalemia (most dangerous period ill-defined; the safest recommendation may be avoidance of this drug)

Nondepolarizing muscle relaxant requirements increased (pharmacodynamic explanation)

5. Ketamine with or without nitrous oxide is often selected as an anesthetic for dressing changes or escharotomies. A volatile anesthetic (often halothane) may be recommended during high-intensity stimulation associated with harvesting the skin graft.

XVI. ELECTRICAL BURN (Table 32-27)

XVII. SEPARATION OF CONJOINED TWINS requires two anesthetic teams and separate anesthetic machines, extensive and invasive monitoring, and consideration of the effect of cross-circulation on responses to drugs. Aggressive efforts are required to maintain normothermia. The need for postoperative support of ventilation is predictable.

Table 32-27. *Characteristics of an Electrical Burn*

Deep tissue injury may be extensive despite limited superficial damage

Cardiac dysrhythmias (cardiopulmonary arrest may have occurred initially, especially with lightening injury)

Renal failure (myoglobin from injured skeletal muscles)

Neurologic complications (direct injury to nerves or subsequent scarring)

Cataract formation a late sequela

Scarring of oral commissures

CHAPTER 33

Physiologic Changes and Disorders Unique to Aging

Aging is accompanied by unavoidable decreases in organ function and by altered responses to drugs (see Stoelting RK, Dierdorf SF. Physiologic changes and disorders unique to aging. In: Anesthesia and Co-Existing Disease. 3rd Ed. New York. Churchill Livingstone, 1993). It is important to recognize that there is not necessarily a correlation between biologic and chronologic age.

I. ORGAN SYSTEM FUNCTION (Table 33-1)

A. Delirium (acute onset of mental confusion) and dementia (Alzheimer's disease) are the two syndromes characterized by global cognitive impairment (Table 33-2). The elderly are susceptible to delirium as a consequence of almost any physical illness (pneumonia, myocardial infarction) or intoxication with even therapeutic doses of commonly used drugs.

B. The ability of the aged heart to increase cardiac output in response to stress may be impaired and vulnerability to drug-induced decreases in myocardial contractility may be increased.

II. PHARMACOKINETICS AND PHARMACODYNAMICS

A. Age-related changes in pharmacokinetics most often manifest as an **increased elimination half-time** of drugs, making the elderly patient vulnerable to cumulative drug effects, especially with repeated doses.

B. Pharmacodynamics depicts the responsiveness of receptors to drugs (decreased to catecholamines and volatile anesthetics, unchanged at neuromuscular junction) in elderly patients.

III. MANAGEMENT OF ANESTHESIA

A. **Preoperative evaluation** of the elderly patient includes consideration of the likely presence of co-existing diseases independent of the reason for surgery and an assessment of concomitant drug therapy (Tables 33-3 and 33-4).

Table 33-1. *Changes in Organ System Function That Accompany Aging*

Decline in central nervous system activity (decreased anesthetic requirements)

Disturbances in sleep pattern (daytime fatigue, sleep apnea syndrome)

Decreased responsiveness of the cardiovascular system to autonomic nervous system stimulation (heart rate slows, blood pressure increases, cardiac output parallels decreased organ requirements)

Deterioration of mechanical ventilatory function (decreased elasticity of lungs) and efficiency of gas exchange (decreased PaO_2)

Decreased renal blood flow and glomerular filtration rate (less able to concentrate urine with fluid deprivation, vulnerable to hyponatremia)

Endocrine dysfunction (diabetes mellitus, subclinical hypothyroidism)

Table 33-2. *Differential Diagnosis of Delirium and Dementia*

	Delirium	**Dementia**
Onset	Sudden	Insidious
Course over 24 hours	Fluctuating with nocturnal exacerbation	Stable
Consciousness	Decreased	Unchanged
Attention	Globally disordered	Usually normal
Hallucinations	Common	Uncommon
Orientation	Impaired	Impaired
Psychomotor activity	Unpredictable	Usually normal
Speech	Often incoherent	Difficulty finding words
Physical illness or drug toxicity	Common	Uncommon

1. Anemia and orthostatic hypotension are common preoperative findings.
2. Evidence of cervical arthritis or of vertebrobasilar arter-

Table 33-3. *Co-Existing Diseases That Often Accompany Aging*

Essential hypertension
Ischemic heart disease
Cardiac conduction disturbances
Congestive heart failure
Chronic pulmonary disease
Diabetes mellitus
Subclinical hypothyroidism
Rheumatoid arthritis
Osteoarthritis

Table 33-4. *Drugs Commonly Prescribed for the Elderly Patient*

Drug	Adverse Effect or Drug Interaction
Diuretics	Hypokalemia Hypovolemia
Digitalis	Cardiac dysrhythmias Cardiac conduction disturbances
Beta antagonists	Bradycardia Congestive heart failure Bronchospasm Attenuation of autonomic nervous system activity
Centrally acting antihypertensives	Attenuation of autonomic nervous system activity Decreased MAC
Tricyclic antidepressants	Anticholinergic effects Cardiac dysrhythmias Cardiac conduction disturbances Increased MAC
Lithium	Cardiac dysrhythmias Prolongation of muscle relaxants
Antidysrhythmic agents	Prolongation of muscle relaxants
Antibiotics	Prolongation of muscle relaxants

Table 33-5. *Induction and Maintenance of Anesthesia in the Elderly Patient*

Decreased anesthetic requirement versus delayed onset

Protection of lungs from aspiration (decreased reactivity of protective upper airway reflexes, high incidence of hiatal hernia)

No evidence that a specific anesthetic drug is preferable

Regional anesthesia acceptable for selected operations in alert patients

ial insufficiency (changes in mental status with head position) is sought.

    B. Preoperative medication may be adequately achieved with a preoperative visit (use of an anticholinergic drug is controversial).

    C. Induction and Maintenance of Anesthesia (Table 33-5)

IV. OSTEOPOROSIS is one of the most important disorders of aging, especially in females. Bones weakened by osteoporosis are vulnerable to fractures with minimal trauma (falls).

V. PROGERIA is characterized by premature aging. Death usually occurs by 25 years of age from congestive heart failure or myocardial infarction. The presence of mandibular hypoplasia and micrognathia may lead to difficulty in management of the upper airway and intubation of the trachea.

Index

Pages numbers followed by f *indicate figures; those followed by* t *indicate tables.*